Memory of
Childhood Trauma

Memory of Childhood Trauma

A Clinician's Guide to the Literature

SUSAN L. REVIERE
Georgia State University

FOREWORD BY JOHN BRIERE

THE GUILFORD PRESS
New York   London

©1996 The Guilford Press
A Division of Guilford Publications, Inc.
72 Spring Street, New York, NY 10012
All rights reserved

Printed in the United States of America

This book is printed on acid-free paper.

Last digit is print number: 9 8 7 6 5 4 3 2 1

Library of Congress Cataloging-in-Publication Data

Reviere, Susan L.
    Memory of childhood trauma: a clinician's guide to the literature / Susan L. Reviere.
        p.   cm.
    Includes bibliographical references and index.
    ISBN 1-57230-109-0 (hardcover). — ISBN 1-57230-110-4 (pbk.)
    1. Adult child abuse victims—Psychology.   2. Autobiographical memory.   3. Recovered memory.   4. Psychic trauma in children.
I. Title.
RC569.5.C55R48   1996
616.85′82239—dc20   96-10813
                                                      CIP

For Gene, Yin, and Yang

*And in appreciation of
Pauline Rose Clance,
Katherine Burge-Callaway,
and Bernhard Kempler*

Foreword

Stated in its most objective terms, the topic of this book should not be that controversial. Trimmed of the sensationalism, media coverage, and adversarial courtroom assertions, the topic seems to involve five relatively straightforward questions: (1) Can someone who was abused as a child somehow not have access to those memories in adulthood? (2) If so, what psychological and/or neurophysiological mechanisms might underlie this process? (3) Are there psychological and social variables that determine the accuracy of those memories if they are recalled at a later point? (4) Are there instances where memory reports are substantially distorted renditions of the original event, or complete confabulations of events that did not occur? And (5) if so, how does this occur?

Unfortunately, because child abuse is, itself, deeply embedded in our culture, because it involves the bestselling combination of sex, violence, and courtroom antics, and because those accused of sexually abusing a child have the right to mount a vigorous defense (regardless of their actual innocence or guilt), this issue has catapulted to the center of a wide public debate. In tandem with this debate has been a polarization of the scientific community. One "side" notes that memory is fallible, and cites or provides laboratory data that recollections (especially by children) can be influenced, distorted, or confabulated under certain circumstances (Ceci & Bruck, 1993; Ceci & Loftus, 1994; Lindsay & Read, 1994; Loftus, 1993). The other "side" points to a growing number of studies of self-reported memory loss and subsequent memory recovery for traumatic events in clinical and nonclinical populations, especially for childhood sexual abuse (Briere & Conte, 1993; Elliott & Briere, 1995; Feldman-Summers & Pope, 1994; Herman & Schatzow, 1987; Williams, 1995), and data that some people known to have experienced sexual abuse in childhood nevertheless deny any recall of such maltreatment later in life (Williams, 1994).

The media have fed this debate, first by sensationalizing court cases involving allegations of "repressed" memory and, later, by producing equally dramatic and one-sided pieces suggesting that most—if not all—reports of recovered memories reflect an epidemic of "false memory syndrome." Therapists who treat those who allege childhood abuse experiences often feel attacked, and frequently become defensive. Accused in the courts and by the media of "implanting" false memories in some of those whom they treat, they worry for their clients and for their own well-being, and wince when confronted with obvious examples of incompetent therapeutic practice by other "abuse-specialized" clinicians. A handful of scientists and clinicians on each side appear over and over again in the courts, asserting with seemingly inevitable conviction that true science and practice supports the position of the client represented by their "side." Other, less polarized, professionals are conspicuously less often hired by lawyers and less frequently interviewed by the media.

And, yet, it is likely that this latter group—peopled by the less emphatic—are closer to the truth. This is because the truth, in this instance, is unlikely to conform to a 5-second sound bite, nor does it provide for compelling and unambiguous court testimony. Instead, it may be closer to the following: It is possible to forget upsetting things as a defense against remaining upset, just as it is possible to remember incorrectly or lie about abuse in the service of some other goal. This means that any given report of recovered memory may be generally accurate, partially accurate, quite distorted, or intentionally false. What science and clinical practice must tell us is what probabilities to assign to each of these options in a given instance, as well as what conditions determine how these probabilities align. It is also quite important that we discover how psychotherapy affects this complex situation: How do we help those who suffer from memories of child abuse while not in some way adversely affecting the accuracy of these memories? If memories are unavailable, but could be made available, is this a good idea? Will it help the client to recover or feel better? If so, when and how should it be done?

Luckily, and apropos of the current book, we have come much farther in the study of these issues than might be apparent from current media coverage. Susan Reviere summarizes in detail the clinical and empirical literature on repression, dissociation, and amnesia, and reviews cognitive, neurophysiological, and trauma perspectives on the encoding, storage, and retrieval of traumatic childhood memories. She organizes these divergent sources of data into a coherent picture, and then devotes two chapters to exploring its clinical implications. Some of this is hard reading, involving as it does technical information on cognitive and neurobiological aspects of memory. Importantly, however, Reviere does not rush to premature closure, nor does she allow the reader to do so. This is by far the most extensive and integrated analysis of traumatic memory available, and does not lend itself to easy answers.

We are in the middle of an exciting, albeit challenging, time. Never before have those who have been abused had such a voice or as much potential opportunity for recovery. As well, never have we, as a society, had to grapple as much with notions of what, exactly, constitutes truth, and how much we can rely on what we (or others) remember as fact. Memory is the moment-by-moment record by which we live our lives, yet we are coming to understand that it is a far more complex and subjective phenomenon than we ever realized. Ultimately, however, rape, abuse, and other violence are not subjective—a given act of sexual victimization cannot be transformed into an interesting scientific or social debate merely because its victim may not have complete access to what happened to him or her. Therein lies the challenge for scientists and practitioners alike: How can we promote justice and healing while, at the same time, accepting the limits of memory and the power of pain to destroy and suppress? As this book demonstrates, this goal is elusive but tremendously worthwhile. I hope that the current volume is a harbinger of things to come, wherein rhetoric declines and the harder work of truly understanding trauma and memory becomes our priority.

JOHN BRIERE

Associate Professor of Psychiatry and Psychology
University of Southern California School of Medicine

REFERENCES

Briere, J., & Conte, J. (1993). Self-reported amnesia for abuse in adults molested as children. *Journal of Traumatic Stress, 6,* 21–31.

Ceci, S. J., & Bruck, M. (1993). Suggestibility of the child witness: A historical review and synthesis. *Psychological Bulletin, 113,* 403–439.

Ceci, S. J., & Loftus, E. F. (1994). "Memory work": The royal road to false memories? *Applied Cognitive Psychology, 8,* 351–364.

Elliott, D. M., & Briere, J. (1995). Posttraumatic stress associated with delayed recall of sexual abuse: A general population study. *Journal of Traumatic Stress, 8,* 629–647.

Feldman-Summers, S., & Pope, K. S. (1994). The experience of "forgetting" childhood abuse: A national survey of psychologists. *Journal of Consulting and Clinical Psychology, 62,* 636–639.

Herman, J. L., & Schatzow, E. (1987). Recovery and verification of memories of childhood sexual trauma. *Psychoanalytic Psychology, 4,* 1–14.

Lindsay, D. S., & Read, J. D. (1994). Psychotherapy and memories of childhood sexual abuse: A cognitive perspective. *Applied Cognitive Psychology, 8,* 281–338.

Loftus, E. F. (1993). The reality of repressed memories. *American Psychologist, 48,* 518–537.

Williams, L. M. (1994). Recall of childhood trauma: A prospective study of women's memories of child sexual abuse. *Journal of Consulting and Clinical Psychology, 62,* 1167–1176.

Williams, L. M. (1995). Recovered memories of abuse in women with documented child sexual victimization histories. *Journal of Traumatic Stress, 8,* 649–673.

Contents

Contents

Introduction:
Defining Trauma

Much has been written in scientific and clinical realms addressing the nature of long-term traumatic memory, but neither
anecdotal clinical impressions nor linear laboratory analogues
sufficiently address the complexity of this issue in a systematic
and integrated manner. The need for clinical and theoretical
clarification of this issue has gathered increased urgency with
the emergence of sociopolitical debate about traumatic memory
both within and outside mental health disciplines.

In both applied and theoretical realms, clinicians are increasingly faced with challenges to commonly held theories and
assumptions concerning memory in adult survivors of early
childhood trauma. The veracity of childhood traumatic memory
is an issue of much controversy, calling up new clinical and
theoretical questions about memory processing, including fresh
reflections on both the psychological and cognitive mechanisms
involved and the nature of historical versus reconstructive articulation of personal history.

Many questions are raised. Are traumatic memories necessarily retained? And if so, can they or must they exist in eidetic
form? To what degree are they distorted, and what factors

account for such distortions? Can traumatic memories be repressed . . . or dissociated? Are repression and dissociation different phenomena, and are either different from suppression? Is the issue one of semantics? Or is there, indeed, a traumatic memory process that is, in any way, different from "normal" memory processes? Are our personal narratives veridical? Or, are they subjectively constructed in such a way that precludes the question of historical reality? This book reviews systematically the various realms of theory and research in this area and integrates the disparate threads into a body of thought applicable to clinical understanding of and intervention with the adult survivor of early trauma.

Before commencing discussion of the specific issues concerning the nature of memory in traumatic childhood experiences, it seems essential to consider the nature of "trauma" per se, as the definition itself may influence the nature of the questions asked, the outcomes produced, and the interpretations offered.

Trauma is defined in various ways that may differ among clinicians and between the clinician and laboratory scientist. On one end of a continuum, the clinician may consider "traumatic" any experience, intrapsychic or external, fantasied or real, that is subjectively felt or labeled as traumatic by the client. Of course, the wide range, subjectivity, and lack of clarity of this definition create significant difficulties for objective study of the phenomenon. On the other end of a continuum are laboratory definitions of trauma such as unpleasantness, task failure, affective intensity, stress, or other "negative" emotional states. While these definitions operate under a loose umbrella of "psychic pain" (which is assumed to be the motivation underlying differential memory responses), their narrowness, variety, and specificity are of questionable clinical utility in the consideration of traumatic states.

Freud (1892a) offers a definition of trauma as "any impression which the nervous system has difficulty in dealing with by means of associative thinking or by motor reaction" (p. 32). He offers further clarification of this definition in describing trauma as a situation that presents the mind with a stimulus too powerful to be dealt with in the normal way (Freud, 1917). Pierre Janet conceptualized trauma similarly, describing as traumatic any experience that overwhelms an individual's ability to take adaptive or effective action (van der Kolk, Brown, & van der Hart, 1989). Although these definitions may be difficult to operationalize, they do begin to capture the complexity and the significance of a clinical notion of trauma by acknowledging that the impact of trauma is such that internal resources are overwhelmed and can create neither meaning nor action in the face of the traumatic experience.

The formal definition of a traumatic stressor in the fourth edition of the *Diagnostic and Statistical Manual of Mental Disorders* (DSM-IV; American Psychiatric Association, 1994) notes the presence of an extreme traumatic event that involves "actual or threatened death or serious injury, or a threat to the physical integrity of self or others" and results in "intense fear, helplessness, or horror" (pp. 427–428). DSM-IV further specifies that these conditions may be created either through the direct experience or witnessing of such an event, or by learning about the "unexpected or violent death, serious harm, or threat of death or injury experienced by a family member or other close associate" (p. 424). Examples of such traumatic events are specified, including military combat, violent personal assault, kidnapping, terrorist attack, disasters, severe accidents, developmentally inappropriate sexual experience, and others.

Two other working definitions of trauma also capture the essence of the phenomenon in a comprehensive manner that offers heuristic utility. McCann and Pearlman (1990) define an experience as traumatic if it "(1) is sudden, unexpected, or non-normative, (2) exceeds the individual's perceived ability to meet its demands, and (3) disrupts the individual's frame of reference and other central psychological needs and related schemas" (p. 10). Similarly, Pynoos and Eth (1985) recognize trauma "when an individual is exposed to an overwhelming event resulting in helplessness in the face of intolerable danger, anxiety, and instinctual arousal" (p. 38).

In these definitions of trauma, the magnitude and degree of arousal, disruption, and helplessness in the client are more clearly articulated. Thus trauma is defined as an extraordinary experience that moves beyond sadness, grief, or the more or less commonplace vicissitudes of living. Trauma involves that from which one cannot escape, either emotionally or physically, or that which causes arousal that exceeds one's ability to cope. In evaluating the intensity and subsequent psychological effects of such experiences, other factors to be considered include the magnitude of the initial physiological response, intensity and chronicity of the trauma, stage of cognitive development at onset of trauma, ego resources, cognitive interpretation, severity of interpersonal loss, length of exposure to trauma, degree of threat and personal injury, and novelty and speed of events (van der Kolk & van der Hart, 1989; van der Kolk et al., 1989).

From this frame of reference, then, the issues concerning related memory processes can be more clearly articulated. Within this frame, however, the issue of memory impairment must be addressed. It is widely accepted among clinicians specializing in the treatment of trauma survivors that adult survivors of severe childhood trauma (and even traumatic experience in adulthood) may enter psychotherapy with some degree of memory impairment for the trauma (e.g., Briere, 1989; Claridge, 1992; Courtois, 1992; Herman & Schatzow, 1987; Levis, 1990). Laub and Auerhahn (1993) state the dilemma cogently, noting that trauma creates a quandary

> between the compulsion to complete the process of knowing and the inability or fear of doing so. . . . The knowledge

of trauma is fiercely defended against, for it can be a momentous, threatening, cognitive and affective task, involving an unjaundiced appraisal of events and our own injuries, failures, conflicts, and losses. During massive trauma, fiction, fantasy, and demonic art can become historical fact; this blurring of boundaries between reality and fantasy conjures up affect so violent that it exceeds the ego's capacity for regulation. . . . Trauma also overwhelms and defeats our capacity to organise it. . . . Our psychological abilities are rendered ineffective. (p. 288)

These authors go on to note various degrees of "encapsulation versus integration" of traumatic experiences in addition to various degrees of ownership of the memories (Laub & Auerhahn, p. 289). At its most basic, traumatic memory impairment may be due to an active, if possibly unconscious, decision of the survivor to inhibit recall in order to titrate the degree of reality that can be tolerated as determined by factors mentioned above. However, just as likely is the possibility that the magnitude of the traumatic experience may have the effect of creating vivid and intrusive memories. Or such arousal may overwhelm the psyche to a degree that the memories are completely unavailable. In fact, memory for traumatic events may fall on a continuum from not knowing to full knowing, with degrees of remembrance depending on dynamic, cognitive, social, and neurological factors in complex interaction. Determining the nature and combinations of such factors presents a significant challenge to understanding fully the phenomenon of memory for trauma. Herein lie the controversy and the issue to be systematically approached.

In the first chapter, repression and dissociation are considered with regard to how these psychological processes are theorized to cause memory impairment in relation to early psychic trauma. Specifically, early theories of Sigmund Freud concerning repression and Pierre Janet concerning dissociation are reviewed. Further, current integrative theories concerning horizontal and vertical consciousness are considered as potential repositories for traumatic memories. The second chapter considers more recent cognitive-behavioral theories concerning the relationship of trauma to the consolidation (or loss) of memories to schemas about self and the world. It has been postulated that traumatic experience is incongruent with safe-world schemas and positive self-schemas, making assimilation impossible. However, accommodation of schemas to the threatening information is not desirable; thus, the traumatic memory may remain unintegrated and, thereby, inaccessible. The third chapter examines the realm of cognitive science in regard to the specific mechanisms and processes of memory such as encoding, long-term retention, and retrieval. Various memory modalities are addressed (verbal, sensory, affective, etc.); specific findings concerning the interaction of traumatic events and memory systems are also reviewed; and developmental issues are explored. The fourth chapter briefly reviews current neurophysiological research relating to trauma and memory. Although much of this work is in its early stages, the findings hold much promise for integration with clinical and cognitive theories in clarifying the issue of traumatic memory. Next, the issue of "truth" is considered in terms of the adult trauma survivor in psychotherapy. Specifically, as the adult survivor of early trauma strives to integrate the traumatic memory in therapy, issues concerning the manner in which the client and therapist reconstruct the client's history takes on primary importance. As such, autobiographical memory is examined in terms of its narrative and/or historical truths in the process of psychotherapy. Finally, conceptual and applied issues in memory work in psychotherapy with adult survivors of early trauma are considered, with special consideration given to the ethics of such therapy work. The last chapter considers research in the field.

Repression and Dissociation

Both historically and currently, the phenomenon of traumatic memory inevitably is considered in relation to the processes of repression and dissociation. Specifically, these concepts have been useful clinical explanations of the memory impairment often observed in trauma survivors. They have also served as the basis for much of the theoretical exploration and empirical research concerned with trauma and memory. Many clinicians are quite comfortable with these terms relative to their heuristic utility in understanding the complex interplay between emotion and memory. Ample clinical and even some laboratory evidence exists to validate the existence of motivated forgetting, perhaps due to repression or dissociation. However, much has been written in refutation of these phenomena as explanations of such forgetting. In fact, certain bodies of laboratory research have failed to demonstrate repression, leading some to question the existence of such a phenomenon (e.g., Holmes, 1990). On both sides of the controversy, these concepts hold a central position in the theoretical, philosophical, and scientific debate concerning traumatic memory; thus it seems essential to understand the nature of repression and dissociation as originally defined and currently understood. From this basis, we can consider the utility of these concepts and the possible mechanisms involved in each.

Early Conceptualizations

REPRESSION

Sigmund Freud is credited with the articulation of the theory of repression. In his early writings on hysterical attacks (1892a), Freud described the process of repression as one in which a patient "intentionally seeks to forget an experience, or forcibly repudiates, inhibits and suppresses" (p. 32). Here, he described a conscious process of refusing to deal with traumatic memories to avoid distress, social stigma, or nervous system incapacitation. He recognized that this refusal would lead to the production of symptoms then referred to as "hysteria." In fact, Freud (1892a) noted that "hysterical patients suffer principally from reminiscences" (p. 40). He first used the term "repression" in a later writing (1892b) in which he noted a deliberate process of motivated forgetting due to the inability of the patient to appropriately "abreact" the traumatic impression (p. 42). In his early writings, Freud made little distinction among the concepts of repression, suppression, and dissociation, and neither in these writings nor in later ones did he stipulate that the process of motivated forgetting necessarily be conscious or unconscious (Erdelyi, 1990).

However, Freud did address the repository for the traumatic memories more specifically. Initially, he differed little from his contemporaries in referring to altered states of consciousness where memories survive with "wonderful freshness and with full affective tone" (1892b, p. 41). At times, he referred to a "second state of consciousness" as "unconscious," as in absent from a patient's "normal state" (1892a, p. 31). Like others, Freud named these altered states "hypnoid states" and referred to their activation as "hysterical attacks" (1892a, pp. 32–33) in which the patient returned to the altered consciousness, stimulated either by exhaustion or by associational triggers. In these states, the trauma was thought to be relived. In referring to this "splitting of consciousness," Freud (1892b) noted that hypnoid states attained differing degrees of psychical organization (p. 44). He described variability in the nature of these states and the degree to which they were accessible to normal consciousness (Erdelyi & Goldberg, 1979). He speculated that these states were not part of normal consciousness per se, because the alteration in state during trauma (caused, in part, by affective intensity) rendered the memory traces, or ideational complexes, unconnected associatively to other memory systems in the consciousness of the patient (1892a, 1892b). In other words, the patient's desire to forget, or not think of, the traumatic material excluded the formation of such associations. It is interesting to note that, at least thus far in his explication of this phenomenon, the descriptions sound much like those of dissociation and dissociated states.

Later in the development of his theory, however, Freud made a departure from his previous descriptions of repression, offering greater clarity in definition and distinguishing it from dissociation. In a 1912 paper, Freud refuted with some disdain the concept of dissociation (or double consciousness) in calling the idea of an "unconscious conscious . . . a gratuitous assumption based on an abuse of the word conscious" (p. 52). He then discussed the process of splitting (i.e., dissociation) in a rather amorphous manner and dismissed it without attempting to explicate or acknowledge the process any further (1912, 1915b). Rather, he focused on further developing his evolving conception of the process of repression.

In his seminal publication, *The Interpretation of Dreams* (1900), Freud discussed repression in terms of the manifestation of unconscious memory traces in dreams, using this as evidence that neither memories nor any other mental contents are ever entirely lost. However, they may be rendered inaccessible to consciousness due to overwhelming affect which, though avoided or repressed, still strives for motor discharge or, at least, "hallucinatory revival," in either dreams or in the reliving of the trauma (p. 644). In his paper on repression, Freud (1915a) further elucidated his concept, defining repression as "the function of rejecting and keeping something out of consciousness" (p. 105) and describing the motivation as avoidance of psychic pain and incapacitation of the ego. In this theory Freud suggested that repressed material continues "to exist, put forth derivatives, and institute connections" (p. 106). However, here still is an implicit suggestion that repression may be a product of conscious intention rather than unconscious processing, offering no clear conceptual distinction between repression and the defensive maneuver of suppression.

Freud described two potential processes of repression, both of which require an ego structure strong enough to hold the unwanted material out of consciousness. In the first, primal repression, the material to be repressed is prevented from entering consciousness at all (Freud, 1915a; Kinston & Cohen, 1986). In other words, the unacceptable content arises from an internal source and is prevented from ever reaching conscious awareness. This idea seems less relevant to external traumatic events than to unacceptable intrapsychic (i.e., id) drives or wishes, such as oedipal sexual fantasies and such. More pertinent to this discussion is Freud's second process, after-expulsion or repression proper, whereby the unacceptable material achieves consciousness briefly and is pushed back into the unconscious in order to ensure the ego's continued integrity (1915a). This type of repression might apply to intrapsychic fantasies or to actual external events, either of which is represented in conscious awareness before being relegated to the irretrievable unconscious. Freud suggested that this process operates by means of two internal "censors," one between unconscious and preconscious realms (with preconscious being a latent form of consciousness), and one between preconscious and conscious realms. Traumatic material can be both pushed from consciousness and pulled from unconsciousness, a degree of force necessary as the material itself most naturally strives toward consciousness and expression (1915b). Freud further clarified this process as a "withdrawal of energic cathexis" (1915a, p. 112), or a withdrawal of the investment of psychic energy, from consciousness or preconsciousness to unconsciousness. He also explained that to achieve consciousness, the traumatic material must be present in both ideational and verbal forms, with one function of repression being the denial of the rejected idea's translation into words or verbal narrative.

In later writings, Freud (1917) again discussed the fact that repressed memories cause symptoms that remit only on reestablishing the connections between the symptoms and the repressed memories. Thus he believed recovery of traumatic memories to be both possible and necessary for healing. From this viewpoint, particularly since repressed material requires significant amounts of intrapsychic energy to ensure its continued inaccessibility to consciousness, the reconnection and reintegration of the unconscious material with the conscious ego are essential to optimal psychic functioning. Specifically, the process of derepression could contribute to smoother psychic functioning, increased availability of psychic energy for other cognitive and emotional tasks, and reduced likelihood of parapraxes, or unexplainable slips of the unconscious material into conscious expression. Thus retrieval of unconscious material became a cornerstone of psychoanalytic theory and practice.

An apt metaphor for Freud's process of recovering memories might be that of an archeological dig (Bonanno, 1990a). Specifically, one starts with symptoms and traces their meaning through layers of history until one finds, usually in the unconscious, the source of the symptom and translates this into verbal consciousness (Freud, 1915a; van der Kolk & van der Hart, 1991). Freud cautioned, however, that surface memories of a seemingly indifferent nature may, in many cases, be "screen memories" of more threatening or traumatic material further below the surface. He felt that these screen memories might be fragments or associations of events or amalgamations of several details available in consciousness or preconsciousness as a compromise between the desire to not know and the push for the material to be known (Freud, 1899).

For Freud, these "memories" might be of actual events or of imagined events. In recanting his seduction theory that the origin of traumatic neurosis was to be found in actual infantile sexual experiences, he posited that infantile sexual wishes and fantasies might also create later symptoms, and once in the unconscious, these may be indistinguishable from real events. This theoretical revision was key in the evolution of Freud's theory. However, for purposes of this discussion, the focus is on the processing of memories for real, not fantasized, experiences.

Both prior to this shift in theory and afterwards, Freud faced questions and challenges regarding the historical truth of the repressed memories of his patients. Although his theory of infantile fantasy, in part, circumvented such questions, he never denied the reality of traumatic experience in some patients and discussed many case studies of recovered memories with corroboration from external sources (Freud, 1892b). Like clinicians today, Freud dealt with challenges that his patients invented memories or that he created traumatic memories iatrogenically. He countered that the distress, reluctance, and disbelief of patients rendered unlikely the possibility of invention, and he noted that he, himself, had experienced neither the inclination nor the ability to induce such ideas in patients (1896). These positions are strikingly similar to arguments being made a century later in response to the debate around recovered memories.

With his theory of repression well articulated and, he believed, well-defended, Freud considered once again the place of dissociation in trauma. In a manuscript left incomplete at the end of his life, Freud (1938) gave credence to dissociation as a valid phenomenon (in addition to repression) in which psychic trauma creates a "rift in the ego" allowing "contrary reactions" that persist as the center point of the split (p. 276). Although this idea was never again expanded, it indicated a possible synthesis in Freud's thinking allowing for both phenomena (van der Kolk & van der Hart, 1991; Bonanno, 1990a).

DISSOCIATION

While Freud's ideas evolved and gained recognition, Pierre Janet conducted systematic observation of more than 5,000 cases to develop a remarkably sophisticated theory of dissociation that is a basis for much thought and research on the phenomenon today (Ellenberger, 1970; Putnam, 1989). In his studies on hysteria, Janet believed dissociation to be the result of traumatic experience that overwhelms the ability to take adaptive action, creating helplessness and causing overwhelming emotions that interfere with verbal understanding and processing (van der Kolk et al., 1989; van der Hart & Friedman, 1989). More specifically, he believed that such traumatic experience causes "pathological diminution and fragmentation of the normal ego" (Nemiah, 1979, p. 316). Janet posited that in normal functioning, the ego maintains the strength and integrity to contain all mental functions, including memories, in an integrated, unified personality dominated by a central ego that sustains awareness of personal identity (Nemiah, 1979; Parkin, 1987). However, in dissociation, this containing function is compromised.

Unlike Freud, who believed motivated forgetting (i.e., repression) to be the function of a relatively well-developed ego, Janet (1892) attributed dissociation to a genetically determined psychic weakness involving either a lack of psychic energy or an inability to utilize this energy (Erdelyi, 1990; Janet, 1892). Such a weakened ego, according to Janet, cannot maintain an integrated unity because of a "narrowing of the field of consciousness incapable of holding all the psychological phenomena" (Janet, 1892, p. 364). Thus "divisions of consciousness" result, provoking "a scission in the continuity of the recollections" and, indeed, in the continuity of the self (1892, pp. 415, 441).

More specifically, Janet (1892) described these divisions of consciousness as abnormal psychological states, or somnambulisms. Such states might vary in complexity from a single image or thought to bodily manifestations to alter personalities (van der Hart & Friedman, 1989). In any case, the patient in a somnambulistic state possesses memories of some form that are isolated from and unavailable in the normal state of consciousness. He referred to these memories as "subconscious fixed ideas" that contain cognitive, affective, and visceral components of the traumatic experience and that serve the purpose of organizing traumatic memories in alternate states of consciousness out of normal conscious awareness (van der Kolk et al., 1989; van der Kolk & van der Hart, 1989). Janet (1892) observed that fixed ideas, while separate from normal consciousness, still influence perceptions, affects, and behaviors and can be expressed as words, actions, somatic responses, or obsessional preoccupations during hysterical attacks, dreams, hypnosis, hallucinations, or "natural somnambulisms" (p. 280).

In explaining the memory impairment in somnambulistic states, Janet maintained that in addition to interference of strong emotions in the memory storage process, a sort of memory phobia also occurs in which the field of consciousness is narrowed in order to avoid the traumatic memory (van der Kolk & van der Hart, 1989). As a result, the mental contents of the alternate states develop outside normal consciousness and are held together by associative connections to the focal fixed idea (i.e., a constellation of traumatic associations). These contents cannot be perceived unless in exactly the same state of consciousness, because the associative network is not connected to the normal state of consciousness (due to avoidance or dissociation). He further noted that the isolation of such memories or mental contents keeps them disconnected from the "complete life" or personal identity of the patient (Janet, 1892, p. 104).

Like Freud, Janet felt that accessing the traumatic memories was key to recovery. The integration of the memories and mental contents of the somnambulistic (or dissociated) states with the normal state of consciousness allows the personal identity again to become continuous and complete. And also like Freud, he observed that the key to such recovery is the transformation of the dissociated traumatic material into a verbal narrative to be integrated with other memories in the life story or personal history of the patient (Parkin, 1987; van der Kolk & van der Hart, 1989; van der Hart, Brown, & van der Kolk, 1989).

SUMMARY: EARLY CONCEPTUALIZATIONS OF REPRESSION AND DISSOCIATION

The similarities and differences in early theories concerning repression and dissociation, can be summarized as follows: In terms of psychological resources or ego strength, repression is thought to involve a strong ego's active, forceful rejection of traumatic material, while dissociation may involve an ego unable to bind or contain various psychic elements in a single, integrated flow of consciousness. Regarding accessibility, repression renders memories irretrievable by any voluntary or conscious control under any circumstances, whereas dissociation retains memories in parallel segregated systems that are available to introspective awareness in certain alternate states of consciousness. In regard to the nature of the processes, repression may be related more to the primary process thinking of the unconscious, where the repressed material becomes indistinguishable from instinctual fantasies; dissociation, however, seems most often to retain a secondary process level of functioning, with fragmented ego states retaining relative ability for reality testing. Theoretically, then, the memories themselves remain intact, clear, and untransformed in dissociation, whereas repressed material may be condensed, disguised, screened, or otherwise distorted. Further, dissociated memories may relate more specifically to traumatic events, whereas repressed memories may involve chronic life stress, trauma, or unconscious fantasies or impulses. The symptoms in overt behavior also vary, with the results of dissociation manifesting as loss of discrete periods of time and repression manifesting as dreams, slips of the tongue, transference reactions, and other parapraxes. Finally, recovery of memory in dissociation is thought to be most often full and rapid in the proper state of consciousness, whereas recovery of repressed memory involves a slow process of accessing deeper and deeper associations and strands of meaning (Erdelyi, 1990; Kihlstrom & Hoyt, 1990; Nemiah, 1979; Spiegel, 1990; Spiegel, Frischholz, & Spira, 1993).

Current Conceptualizations

Most current conceptualizations of repression and dissociation are clearly built on the early theories of Freud and Janet whose insights into these phenomena demonstrated remarkable foresight. However, many current theories of repression and dissociation strive for integration, attributing traumatic memory inhibition to a combination of repressive and dissociative processes impinging on a consciousness that includes both horizontal and vertical components. This spatial metaphor specifies a topography of the mind consisting of a horizontal component divided into conscious and unconscious layers by a repression barrier and a vertical component composed of separate psychological units or subsystems divided by alterations in consciousness (Beahrs, 1982; Fromm, 1992; Hilgard, 1977). Each of these components will be considered.

REPRESSION AND HORIZONTAL SPLITS

Theoretically, repression is thought to be the mechanism by which the horizontal division between the conscious and unconscious realms is established and maintained. With regard to trauma, repression involves an expulsion of the unwanted traumatic memory from consciousness, although the continuity of consciousness remains intact (van der Kolk & van der Hart, 1991). Theoretically, the traumatic material has been allowed enough conscious processing for adequate encoding to take place, but repression causes this information to be blocked at the retrieval stage (Terr, 1994). Thus two basic layers of consciousness exist in repression: normal consciousness and the unconscious. (Freud's original topographical model included a preconscious that could be considered a latent form of consciousness.) Repressed material is pushed downward into the unconscious where it remains inaccessible to volitional retrieval under any circumstances. Its existence is inferred from symbolic, indirect, or affective expressions or from symptoms that seem incomprehensible and, in some cases, ego-alien.

Repression may cause amnesia primarily for episodic memory (which involves explicit memory for personal events), but not for semantic memory (which involves procedural knowledge of the world). Further, affect associated with the traumatic experience is thought to remain in consciousness (Vaillant, 1990). Thus, in a traumatic experience, the episodic content may be rendered inaccessible, while the procedural memories or affects, such as inappropriate attributional styles or irrational fears, remain intact without conscious awareness of how such pathogenic knowledge or feelings were acquired (Erdelyi, 1990; Kihlstrom & Hoyt, 1990; Nemiah, 1979; Spiegel, 1990; Vaillant, 1990).

Once removed from consciousness, the episodic memory lost to repression may become inextricably mired and transformed by unconscious content that includes fantasies, instincts, wishes, and fears. As such, it may be entangled in a process of thinking that is fantasy-based, nonlinear, and nonrational (i.e., primary process thinking) (Spiegel et al., 1993; Nemiah, 1979). Thus unlike normal forgetting, repression, because it is a defensive process, may lead to greater distortion and may leave memories irretrievable even with the cues that might reinstate normally decaying memories (Terr, 1994).

Although repressed memories may be unavailable, the process of repression may occur without interfering significantly with the continuity of conscious experience. While portions of personal memory may be inaccessible, a basic continuity in sense of self, others, and the world in day-to-day experience remains intact in repression. Thus in childhood, the horizontal split of repression may not interfere with the development of a cohesive self and may allow unhindered development of a system of a relatively continuous memory for personal history (i.e., autobiographical memory) situated spatially and temporally.

Beyond this current conceptualization, reminiscent of Freud's original theories, what is clear is that while the existence of the phenomenon of repression is acknowledged by many, neither the exact nature of this process nor its differentiation from dissociation (or even suppression) is clearly understood or agreed upon. Even Freud over the course of his many writings discussed the process of repression in myriad ways, often leaving the reader unclear as to the precise nature of the process as distinct from other defensive processes and, indeed, often using repression as a metaexplanation for a class of related psychological defenses (Singer & Sincoff, 1990). Therefore, much is unresolved both theoretically and empirically about the nature of this phenomenon.

DISSOCIATION AND VERTICAL SPLITS

Current clinical theories of dissociation are, perhaps, better developed than those of repression, although dissociation, too, has been the subject of myriad definitions. Dissociation has been variably described as a process that creates semi-independent subsystems that are neither consciously accessible nor integrated with conscious memory, identity, or volition; an alteration in consciousness involving the disconnection of some aspects of self or environment; or a defensive maneuver used to ward off physical or emotional pain resulting in a lack of personality integration (Cardeña, 1994). Returning to the spatial metaphor, dissociation has likewise been related to vertical components in the mind. From a clinical or personality standpoint, these components, or psychological subsystems, are coexisting constellations of cognitive elements, such as affect, thought, and memory, that are kept more or less separate by interruptions in a sense of conscious continuity. Further, dissociation in this sense can be thought of as involving that which is not available to voluntary conscious awareness. In other words, that which should ordinarily be accessible to or integrated in an individual's consciousness and sense of a historically extended self is neither available nor integrated (Cardeña, 1994). These psychological subsystems may be thought of as roughly akin to, but perhaps involuntary forms of, schemas, roles, ego states, or moods (Beahrs, 1982; Cardeña, 1994).

Although several current theories, such as hypnotic susceptibility (i.e., autohypnosis) and neurobiology, are useful in understanding dissociation, perhaps the most comprehensive and inclusive theory explains dissociation in terms of states of consciousness. In general terms, dissociation is best understood as a discontinuity in consciousness attributable to development of discrete states, with "state" being defined as "a recurrent interactive organization of consciousness that organizes or structures perception, cognition, and behavior" (Putnam, 1990, p. 122). Such states are thought to maintain some degree of internal coherence discrete from other states. Transitions between states are associated with "rapid, nonlinear changes in (1) affect, (2) attention and cognition, (3) retrieval of memories and access to learned skills, (4) autonomic physiology, and (5) sense of self" (Putnam, 1989, p. 423). A further implication is that the ego functioning within each vertical state remains more or less intact in terms of higher cognitive functioning and rational, linear, reality-based thinking (i.e., secondary process thinking) (Nemiah, 1979). Thus, the memorial content of each parallel system remains associatively connected and intact without significant distortion when in that specific state (Spiegel et al., 1993). As such, the dissociated states of consciousness are usually marked with a strong central affect, a specific cognitive style, a set of memories and behaviors that are state-dependent, and a state-dependent sense of self.

In fact, Putnam (1989) and others understand dissociation largely as an extreme form of state-dependent learning and memory processing. From this model, dissociation is conceptualized on a continuum. One end of this continuum involves "normal" dissociation (e.g., daydreaming or absorption in a book or movie) in which a fluid sense of experience remains basically intact. At the other extreme, dissociation involves states that are separate, discontinuous, and, in some cases, mutually exclusive (Putnam, 1990, 1991, 1993). It is at this end of the dissociative continuum that dissociation is clearly defined as pathological, as it involves alterations in phenomenal or subjective experience related to a disconnection or disengagement within the self or between self and the environment (Cardeña, 1994). Thus, dissociation is a complex psychological process common not only in psychopathology but also in normative human development and experience.

Developmental research relevant to this matter suggests that physiological state changes in infants underlie changes in states of consciousness that may be the basic building blocks of human behavior. Specifically, the "normal" experience of infants and children is thought to involve a predominance of marked state changes that produce a discontinuity in a child's experience of self and the world. In normative development, parents structure the child's environment to titrate stimulation and facilitate self-regulation through soothing rituals. With this parental intervention, the discrete states are bridged over time in such a way that shifts between them are blended into a more continuous, stable experience of the world and of the self.

In individuals with early experiences of trauma, however, stimulation and attendant arousal states may be augmented rather than titrated, and the developmentally appropriate blending of states is thought to be disrupted such that abrupt state transitions continue, discontinuous experience predominates, and processes of memory and identity are disturbed (Putnam, 1990; van der Kolk & van der Hart, 1989; Waites, 1993). Thus, for a child who has experienced trauma, the childhood propensity for dissociation, normally decreased through maturation, is more fully developed and is retained in adult behavior as a means of moderating stimulation and organizing coping (Putnam, 1991; Waites, 1993). However, once the trauma has ended, dissociation is neither necessary nor adaptive, as the continued existence of discrete states and discontinuous shifts between them interfere with integrative functioning and continuity of memory, identity, and sense of self and others.

While these ideas suggest a developmental role for multiple states and dissociative processes in normative experience, there is less focus on and explication of the mechanisms underlying the blending of states or the disruption of such a process. Certainly, much like Janet, some consider continuity of experience to define normative functioning and discontinuity to be the result of some imposing force or process upon a compromised ego structure, such as the erection of amnestic barriers within a normatively continuous, unified ego. Others consider that the mind is normatively discontinuous, with continuity simply an illusion created by conscious awareness.

From the first point of view, however, normative experience is continuous, with dissociative processes pathologically disrupting the continuity. Here the focus is on this loss of integrative functioning caused by dissociation rather than on the existence of dissociative states of consciousness per se. Dissociation, from this perspective, is an inborn biopsychological predisposition, utilized defensively and best understood by its results: splitting off from consciousness the psychological processes of behavior, affect, sensation, and knowledge (the BASK model) that are normally integrated in one's experience of self and the world (Braun, 1990). Dissociation thus may involve "a defensive disruption in the normally occurring connections among feelings, thoughts, behavior, and memories" (Briere, 1992, p. 36). The memory impairment here tends to involve, like repression, primarily episodic memory, with semantic or procedural knowledge remaining intact. In any case, such a disruption may be caused by a withdrawal of attention during traumatic experience that may attenuate sensory input and interfere with the encoding, storage, and assimilation of the memory into the normal flow of consciousness (Braun, 1990; Terr, 1994; Briere, 1992). This attentional withdrawal may serve the functions of experiential disengagement from overwhelming circumstances and conservation of physical and psychological resources during inescapable trauma (Cardeña, 1994). The attendant loss in integrative processing may be related to a dysregulation of awareness for the normal, ongoing mediation between simultaneous cognitive and perceptual processes. Thus, splits between states or networks of meaning or splits between affect and content are produced, resulting in a split-off, parallel relationship to normal conscious awareness (Spiegel, 1990).

With continuous exposure to trauma, the disruption in the process and functioning of consciousness may result in a chaining of trauma-related episodic memories and associated response patterns into functionally separate divisions of experience defined by some degree of memory impairment (e.g., amnestic barriers) and containing isolated sets of affects and memories that have become segregated (Braun, 1990; Spiegel, 1990). Although these parallel vertical systems may be mutually exclusive and transiently denied access to a single conscious control, their contents remain available to state-specific introspective awareness (Kihlstrom & Hoyt, 1990; Spiegel, 1990).

Other conceptualizations, not entirely dissimilar, assign greater prominence to a normative discontinuity in mental functioning (Hilgard, 1977, 1992, 1994; Woody & Bowers, 1994). Here, the architecture of the mind involves a multiplicity of processes with coexisting levels of control, all subsumed and coordinated under a higher conscious functioning (Woody & Bowers, 1994). Specifically, the mind is composed of separate subsystems, or cognitive structures, handling various cognitive processes simultaneously. These cognitive structures are hierarchically organized and monitored by an executive function (or central processor) that allows varying degrees of submonitoring by each of the components for its own processing (Hilgard, 1992, 1994; Kihlstrom, 1992). In normal functioning, this structure allows an individual to organize, process, plan, and evaluate on various levels simultaneously, with the cognitive structures in communication with each other and with the central processor. However, in dysfunctional processing, these connections are somehow impaired, the relationship of the executive control system to consciousness is altered, and the "illusory" sense of a unified consciousness is disrupted (Hilgard, 1992, p. 16; Woody & Bowers, 1994). Specifically, the various cognitive structures are less integrated, and although the cognitive structures may continue processing, they do so in the absence of a feedback loop with other cognitive structures or with the executive function (Hilgard, 1992; Kihlstrom, 1992). Thus the parallel processing that normally operates under the umbrella of continuity offered by executive control is exposed by the removal or alteration of that control function (Woody & Bowers, 1994). These ideas have been applied to empirically validated phenomena, including familiar neuropsychological and clinical phenomena such as alexia without agraphia, expressive aphasia without receptive aphasia, implicit perception, multiple personality disorder, and others (Kihlstrom, 1992).

In general, then, the discontinuity theories posit various processes that occur simultaneously but appear to be unified and continuous due to the organization provided by consciousness itself. However, these ideas leave unexplained the observed internal coherence of the states noted in the state model. If dissociation is simply a function of a weakened control function, then cognitive processes would be less integrated, but the cognitive system would not necessarily produce the constellations of personality-like states of consciousness, each with its own more or less integrated functioning.

Despite distinct theoretical positions on the phenomenon of dissociation, most likely is the probability that dissociation, like most other mental processes, is multiply determined by numerous factors in varying combinations. It may be that both the continuity and discontinuity models are, in certain aspects, accurate in describing the process and mechanisms of dissociation. It is quite likely that various cognitive processes operate in parallel. It is also likely that higher cognitive processes involving the functions of conscious awareness impose a certain continuity to experience as well as a sense of the self as stable. Dissociation may involve, in general, a dysregulation in a supraordinate conscious control system. The results of this dysregulation may include both some loss in the sense of continuity normally imposed upon various mental processes (such as in the BASK model) and some heightened ability for these processes to then serve as focal points for the adaptive and compensatory development of constellations that come to include other cognitive elements (as in the state model). In any case, the various current conceptualizations of dissociation, while well articulated, still require some degree of integration in order to enhance understanding of both clinical and experimental observations of dissociative processes.

Summary: Repression and Dissociation

Currently, as historically, many descriptions of the nature of repression and dissociation are highly similar, with distinctions often drawn in theory concerning the topography of consciousness or the cognitive mechanisms of action, which are reviewed in subsequent chapters. Further, while current thinking acknowledges both horizontal and vertical layers of consciousness, many explain their coexistence, and thus their distinctions, by concluding that the process of repression functions to manage both internally derived unacceptable material (e.g., impulses, wishes, aggressive fantasies) and external stressors, while the process of dissociation serves primarily to manage external trauma (van der Kolk & van der Hart, 1991). Or it may be that both are part of a process in which a complex memory with its various sensory, cognitive, and emotional associations is fragmented, with some components repressed (by way of one of several specific cognitive mechanisms) and others available in alternate states of consciousness (Beahrs, 1982; Erdelyi, 1990; Singer & Sincoff, 1990).

The lack of full integration of both processes is one failure of the horizontal–vertical consciousness model. A clear explanation of if and how traumatic memories per se can be both dissociated and repressed at once remains to be fully articulated. Further, the theoretical (and clinical) elaboration of these ideas has yet to integrate adequately the role of cognitive processes well known to memory researchers. As consciousness and memory are processes, rather than actual spatial structures, a fuller comprehension may emerge in exploring the complexity of these processes and the possible mechanisms underlying them.

Trauma and Cognitive Schemas

Schema theory is, in a sense, a theory of memory and thus may be used to understand some of the memory processes in traumatic experience. Some writers relate schema theory to the concepts of repression and dissociation, proposing models linking the memory impairment often seen in trauma with an underlying motivational mechanism related to the preservation of schematic integrity. Thus schema theory may provide a bridge between dynamic conceptualizations of traumatic memory and the relationship of these conceptualizations to cognitive processes. Before considering the details of these ideas, however, the concept of schema and ideas concerning schematic development must be clearly articulated as they will be discussed herein.

Schema Defined

The concept of schema, as introduced by Bartlett (1932), is defined as a general knowledge structure that includes principal attributes, the relationships among these attributes, and specific exemplars (Singer & Salovey, 1993). According to Bruhn (1990), schemas are "expectations, rules, or axioms derived from past experience that the individual maintains about himself, others, and the world" (p. 49). McCann and Pearlman (1990) define the concept similarly, adding that schemas represent general knowledge about objects, situations, and events; organize reality; and provide realistic expectations that guide characteristic ways of attending, remembering, interpreting, and responding to the world. They note that schemas are cognitive manifestations (with affective valences) of psychological needs such as trust, safety, power, esteem, independence, and intimacy. Horowitz (1991) further specifies that schemas are summaries of experiences represented in generalized, modular forms that serve as templates for organization of incoming information. He and others (e.g., Bartlett, 1932; Mandler, 1983; Piaget, 1970; Schachtel, 1959) suggest that the existence of cognitive schemas enables rapid perception and expectation in responding to the vast stimuli presented on a moment-to-moment basis in both internal and external worlds.

The study of schematic processing conducted by cognitive psychologists provides a basis for many of the related clinical observations and theories. An expansive body of research has considered the economy of processing afforded by the availability of schematic networks. Such "top-down, or conceptually driven, processing" affects perception from its very earliest stages, as schemas engender interactive processing that is imbued with schematic knowledge and expectations (Mandler, 1983, p. 454). Specifically, percepts that activate related schemas are encoded more rapidly, remembered more accurately, and elaborated inferentially on the basis of representative or typical exemplars. In addition, schematic expectations may influence which data are encoded and retained (see studies by Mandler and colleagues, cited in Mandler, 1983). Further, anomalous or "low-probability" data are identified less rapidly than data consistent with schematic expectations; however, once identified, more time and attention are dedicated to processing the details of the anomaly in a sort of "bottom-up," or data-driven, processing (Mandler, 1983, pp. 454, 456). With experience and maturity, the increased processing of schematically inconsistent stimuli may lead to improvements in memory for such stimuli as well (Farrar & Goodman, 1990; Mandler, 1983). In general, schemas are understood to be integrated holistic matrices of information that represent general knowledge structures rather than collections of individual episodes. Further, they are temporally, causally, and hierarchically organized in increasingly detailed levels that may include optional or alternative paths of expectation (Bauer, 1995; Hudson, 1986, 1993).

Beahrs (1982) compares the concept of schema to the general concept of states of consciousness, describing both as discrete mental units that are separated by boundaries from other units and that have characteristic features over an extended period of time. He notes that such mental units (i.e., schemas) serve as organizing principles for the psyche. Horowitz (1988, 1991) adds that schemas are organized as a repertoire of subschemas coordinated, more or less, by a supraordinate schema that provides predictability and continuity to a "multiply stable" system (1988, p. 31). At any given time in such a system, one of the subschemas, most likely a self-schema, is the dominant referent for organizing experience, perception, thought, mood, action, and memory (Horowitz, 1991; Singer & Salovey, 1991). This description of schemas is consistent with theories of dissociation specifying substructures subsumed under a central control mechanism.

Again, these clinically based conceptualizations are consistent with cognitive research suggesting that schemas are hierarchically organized with the more specific and limited schemas embedded in ever-larger, supraordinate schemas. Likened to a tree diagram, hierarchically organized schemas may parse goals, subgoals, and actions within an episode, with the most general information at the top of the structure and the most detailed and specific at the bottom. Recall of a single node of the structure is presumed theoretically to cue retrieval of information nested beneath (Bauer, 1995; Hudson, 1986, 1993). These hierarchical matrices include not only detail at each level but also information regarding relationships between various levels. This degree of hierarchical embeddedness may contribute to the importance of context in both recognition and retrieval (Mandler, 1983; Neisser, 1986).

Schema Development

As with most other psychological systems, schemas begin to develop early in life as a child's psychological needs achieve increasing clarity and differentiation and as experiences are repeated and gradually organized for purposes of comprehension and generalization (Hudson, 1993; Mandler, 1983; McCann & Pearlman, 1990; Nelson, 1988). Cognitive psychologists have found that initially schematic organization centers primarily on general information (Hudson, 1993). Mandler (1983) notes that categorization is an innate tendency of early infancy when the infant learns to categorize objects at a basic level, most likely on the basis of perceptual characteristics and functional relations to self. In this early phase of schematic development, schema–congruent information is incorporated, while divergent information is either absorbed as an elaboration or ignored (this process has been referred to as schema confirmation and deployment) (Farrar & Goodman, 1990; Goodman & Golding, 1983; Neisser, 1986). As a result, early in the developmental process, the hierarchical complexity of schemas of young children is limited, rendering the schemas less elaborated and, therefore, "flatter" than those of older children and adults (Bauer, 1995, p. 56). Thus younger children may not have available the retrieval cues provided by the hierarchical organization of complex events (Bauer, 1995; Hudson, 1993).

However, with continued experience, these general schemas continue to differentiate and grow in structural complexity, with "changes in detail, elaboration, and even cohesiveness . . . leading to quantitative improvements in encoding and memory" (Mandler, 1983, p. 454). As experience accumulates over time, schemas continue development and modification through minute calibrations that maintain consistency between expectations (i.e., schemas) and reality. These calibrations involve the processes of assimilation and accommodation. Assimilation integrates incoming information into existing schematic meaning systems, while accommodation requires the schemas themselves to make slight shifts in order to represent reality accurately. For accommodation to occur, however, the anomalous experience must be sufficiently powerful and compelling and must create only moderate levels of affective arousal (Bruhn, 1990; Erdelyi, 1990; McCann & Pearlman, 1990). Otherwise, the incoming perceptions may be either unattended, unintelligible, avoided, or simply excluded from the schematic memory system. In most instances, both assimilation and accommodation occur at a level of unconscious or preconscious processing, allowing automatic, relatively continuous adaptations to self and world (Mandler, 1983; van der Kolk & van der Hart, 1989).

Development requires an equilibration that involves a balancing of assimilative and accommodative processes. This equilibration process maintains balance between organism and environment such that both are experienced as stable and consistent (Fine, 1990). Thus as schemas develop, they orient a growing child to self and world, giving a sense of predictability and continuity that allows for adaptive generalization (Fine, 1990; Piaget, 1970). The primary motivation in the organization of experience and memory becomes the maintenance of identity, continuity, and meaning (Ulman & Brothers, 1988).

Schemas and Memory

In general, memory is most likely composed of schemas relating to self and world rather than of specific, isolated traces or images (Bartlett, 1932; Bruhn, 1990). Schemas can be thought of as networks of information and meaning about specific stimulus domains that compose the memory system. Specific details of discrete events may be embedded in the larger categorical matrix of meaning (Barclay, 1986; McCann & Pearlman, 1990). According to this theory, most memories of one's history are reconstructions of episodic events based on schemas that provide a consistent frame for the experiences of an individual's life (Barclay, 1986; Bartlett, 1932; Neimeyer & Metzler, 1994). Consistent with this view, cognitive research has shown that perceptions tend to be recalled schematically; even when the perceptual input is disorganized, schemas may bias recall in terms of distortions that organize the disorganized percepts canonically (Hudson, 1986; Mandler, 1983). While such reconstructive processes of schematic expectancies can aid recall by providing cues for retrieval, this tendency can, at times, lead to distortions in memory, as the schematic inference biases memory toward the expected (Farrar & Goodman, 1990; Hudson, 1986; Mandler, 1983; Reyna, 1992).

Janet's work very clearly addressed this idea in considering that memory consists of experiences organized and categorized according to existing schemas. In fact, Janet suggested that the memory system maintains continuity and coherence by utilizing these schemas in this way (van der Kolk et al., 1989). In an interpretation of Janet, van der Kolk and van der Hart (1991) describe the memory system as "the central organizing apparatus of the mind, which categorizes and integrates all aspects of experience and automatically integrates them into ever enlarging and flexible meaning schemes" (p. 426). Thus, for an experience to be retained in memory, Janet (1892) suggested that it must be connected or synthesized to a "mass" or "ensemble" of ideas or remembrances, resulting in "psychological assimilation," which he believed to be the key to the psychology of memory (p. 103). He considered memory a creative act in which experiences are assimilated and transformed toward compatibility with existing schemas.

Likewise, both early and more recent cognitive theorists have suggested that a memory system based on schemas constructs highly personalized memories that accentuate schema-consistent details and minimize schema-inconsistent details (e.g., Bartlett, 1932; Farrar & Goodman, 1990; Mandler, 1983; Neisser, 1986). In this sense, schemas are apperceptive screens, with both intellective and emotional aspects, that bias perception toward an active, creative construction of memory (Barclay, 1986; Bruhn, 1990; Horowitz, 1991; Neimeyer & Metzler, 1994). In fact, Barclay (1986) posits that "memories are largely reconstructions aimed at preserving the essential integrity of existing self-structures" (p. 97). This may, in part, explain the fact that schemas are notably perseverant, perhaps in the service of efficiency and continuity, despite conflicting information (Bonanno, 1990b; Singer & Salovey, 1991).

This theory suggests, then, that especially early in development, the memory system should retain events that support existing schemas in the process of schema confirmation. Inconsistent experiences may be disregarded early in schematic development, leaving them unavailable for later recall; however, once schemas are adequately formed and deployed in the service of perception and prediction, an anomalous experience may either be noted as distinctive or incorporated through transformation of the experience to fit the schema or accommodation of the schema to include the experience. In either case, memorial representation in some form should be retained (Barclay, 1986; Erdelyi, 1990; Hudson, 1986; Neisser, 1986). These ideas are supported by research with children demonstrating that older children are better able to recall distinctive events than are younger children who primarily attend to generalized common-alities in experience (Bauer, 1995; Farrar & Goodman, 1990; Fivush & Hamond, 1990).

Schematic memory processing allows coherence and consistency in experiencing the world and enables prepared and adaptive responses to a wide variety of situations. Thus schematic memory targets for storage the data with the greatest potential adaptive value in terms of current coping and future problem solving (Bruhn, 1990). This may, however, render the earliest of episodic memories unavailable for recall.

Schemas and Trauma

As schemas evolve and develop over time, most individuals develop and maintain general, supraordinate themes or assumptions that provide a thread of continuity throughout development and upon which specific schemas are built. These assumptions include basic beliefs about one's worthiness, invulnerability, and safety, in addition to beliefs that the world is just, benevolent, meaningful, and controllable (Janoff-Bulman, 1989). Such expectations ensure the predictability of experience and the regulation of arousal in the face of anomalous experience. In a lifetime without trauma, these assumptions may remain largely unquestioned and unchallenged, and development of schemas will proceed in small, gradual, deliberate, and predictable changes that leave the overall structure of the system stable and coherent (Janoff-Bulman, 1989).

Traumatic experience, however, may provide a direct challenge, rendering basic assumptions and the accompanying schemas obsolete. As traumatic experience is most often profoundly discrepant with existing schematic beliefs and expectations about self in the world, neither assimilation nor accommodation are tolerable options.

Past experience provides little guidance, as trauma presents anomalous data of considerable salience too powerful to ignore. The repetitive life experiences that form schemas often do not include significant trauma, so the schemas provide neither a frame for understanding traumatic experience nor a basis for adaptive action (similar to Janet's ideas concerning trauma and dissociative processing). Particularly since schemas tend to organize perceptual input, traumatic experience may create emotional and cognitive confusion and disorientation that paralyze an individual's ability to respond adaptively.

Accommodation of existing schemas to traumatic data may portend a "catastrophic change" that threatens decompensation, as the most basic human assumptions of worthiness, safety, trust, and predictability are challenged (Janoff-Bulman, 1989, p. 121; Kinston & Cohen, 1986). The salience of and provision of stability afforded by these basic assumptions, along with the need to maintain equilibrium, safety, and emotional modulation, provide powerful motivational factors for leaving the traumatic experience unassimilated and the schemas unaccommodated. Those who do manage over time to accommodate schemas to the traumatic information may experience a loss in regard to basic assumptions previously held. Specifically, they perceive self more negatively, perceive the world more malevolently, and report higher levels of depression (Janoff-Bulman, 1989).

Laub and Auerhahn (1993) discuss traumatic experience, schemas, and psychological functioning, noting that

> trauma overwhelms and defeats our capacity to organize it: facing real threats of massive aggression, our psychological abilities are rendered ineffective. Massive aggressions's pervasive, deconstructive impact on the cultural and psychological assumptions governing our lives often results in cognitive and affective paralysis, from whose vantage point we can only relate to the events as if they had not happened. . . . Knowing these events, making sense of them, putting

them in the order of things, seems like an insurmountable
(and yet unavoidable) task. (p. 288)

The attempt to resolve this crisis of meaning may result in
self-blame which allows higher levels of perceived control,
reinterpretation of the trauma in a positive light (in order to
leave schemas intact), denial, or intrusive and recurring thoughts
about the trauma. Or the individual dealing with trauma may
exhibit a biphasic response, alternating between denial and
intrusion of the traumatic images. Horowitz (1986) suggests that
material that cannot be assimilated immediately into existing
schemas may be held in an "active memory" store that initiates
repetition of the traumatic contents until cognitive processing
(i.e., assimilation/accommodation) is complete (p. 94). During
this repetition/intrusion phase, intense emotions may be evoked
as old schemas are being confronted with unacceptable new
information. In response, a denial phase may be initiated by
cognitive controls that are activated to titrate emotional stimulation and prevent decompensation (Horowitz, 1986, 1991;
McCann & Pearlman, 1990). These controls—which include
choice of mode of representation, locus, time orientation (immediate or long-term), topic, activation level, problem solving
versus reverie, and so forth—may inhibit the path from active
memory storage to representation and processing, and thus this
control process may be responsible for some degree of memory
impairment or distortion.

The optimal outcome of this "completion tendency"
process is the integration of the traumatic experience with
updated, adaptive schemas. However, one outcome of the biphasic response pattern may be "stable defensive distortion" in
which excessive use of controls interrupts information processing, changes the state of the person, and prevents completion
(Horowitz, 1986, p. 86). The memories then may be denied
meaningful conscious awareness because they are not integrated

into schematic memory and thus have no cognitive representation available to voluntary conscious recall. The effects of this outcome include a continuation of periodic uncontrolled intrusion alternating with numbing, memory impairment, dissociation, and inability to integrate the new experience into a life narrative (Horowitz, 1991).

Traumatic Experience in Childhood Schema Development

If trauma is encountered during childhood at a time when schemas and beliefs about the self and world are forming, traumatic experience may interfere with development of supraordinate, general schemas that create a sense of continuity in self, memory, and meaning. Particularly in an environment of chronic trauma, the predictability and stability of experience necessary for the formation of adaptive schemas may be absent, disrupting schema formation at all levels. The distorted schemas of a young survivor of chronic trauma may be defensive attempts to organize a chaotic world (Horowitz, 1991, 1988; Fine, 1990).

Such distortions may disrupt the ability of the developing child to learn and generalize new information effectively, further affecting processes of memory (Fine, 1990). In addition, early trauma may affect adversely the ability of the child to make future assimilations and accommodations and thus may reduce cognitive and behavioral flexibility, impairing the child's ability for adaptation. Specifically, as the traumatized individual leaves key memories unassimilated, later events may not be appropriately interpreted. The survivor then may experience disruption in the ability to interpret reality in terms of existing schemas, failing to build on a personal narrative and to develop a capacity for flexible adaptive action. This disruption in the ongoing ability to adjust schemas to current reality leaves the individual less likely to be able to adapt (van der Kolk et al., 1989).

Further, Schachtel (1947), and later Bruhn (1990), posit that children encode events in preverbal and early verbal forms incompatible with mature cognitive schemas. In addition, the child's immature capabilities for language, thought, and affect modulation may prevent verbal representation. In a child with early chronic trauma, traces of the traumatic experiences may survive only as loose constellations of unintegrated, fragmented percepts, if at all (Laub & Auerhahn, 1993; McCann & Pearlman, 1990). Thus not only may the child have a limited ability to make sense of trauma for incorporation into organized memory; the early experience, even if encoded into some form of early schematic memory, is possibly unintelligible to the adult whose schemas have equilibrated over time.

Schemas, Repression, and Dissociation

If traumatic experience defies a child's ability to understand, categorize, and assimilate, and if accommodation poses a threat too great, memory for traumatic events may be impaired. Thus, the motivation behind "motivated forgetting" may relate to the preservation of self, stability, and safety afforded by intact, coherent, and consistent psychological schemas with attendant modulation in emotional states (Bonanno, 1990b). An integration of schema theory with theories of repression and/or dissociation may provide fuller understanding. Kinston and Cohen (1986) note that repression can occur where psychic structure (i.e., schematic understanding) is absent. In the absence of such structure, which provides organization and meaning, traumatic experience cannot be represented or encoded in any mature, meaningful way. Thus while fragmented sensory impressions, stereotyped actions, physiological reactions, images, and affects may be loosely retained, these all are "prerepresentational." The integrated memory is lost to repression. (Note, however, that this idea excludes the notion of repression as, necessarily, an active forceful expulsion.) McCann and Pearlman (1990) echo this suggestion, discussing the status of memories as either "repressed or accessible, whole or fragmented, tolerable or distressing, intrusive or avoided" (p. 204) depending on the degree of disturbance in core schemas and underlying needs and assumptions. Bruhn (1990) further specifies that memories may be repressed if the individual experiencing trauma is overwhelmed and emotionally unprepared to process such experience or, in general, if events are significantly inconsistent with current schemas. He notes that if growth or preparation occur, however, the memories may be brought into conscious awareness spontaneously. The assumption here, of course, is that the memories unable to be integrated with existing schemas are left unrepresented, moved into the sphere of the unconscious, irretrievable by will, and unavailable in conscious awareness.

Dissociation is, perhaps, more fully articulated as the process of memory impairment stimulated by incompatibility of trauma with existing schemas (Beahrs, 1982; van der Kolk et al., 1989). Janet (1892) first discussed this idea, clearly positing that traumatic experience, in order to be known, must be attached to other memories (e.g., schemas). Otherwise, while the isolated memory processes of "conservation" and "reproduction" (analogous to encoding and retrieval) are intact, a lack of synthesis suppresses the assimilation of memories into the existing personality. He notes "memory is only the preservation of a synthesis previously made; it is plain that memory will not exist when the synthesis has not yet been effected or when it is but half effected and remains unstable and fragile" (1892, p. 108).

Janet (1892) specifies that the memory is dissociated and describes the memory impairment as a disturbance in assimilation. In fact, he notes that "hysterical amnesia is nothing else than a simple amnesia of assimilation" (p. 104), referring to the incompatibility of traumatic experience with existing schemata,

Janet's term for schemas. In order to achieve consciousness, a memory must become part of a "unified memory" of all psychological facets of a particular experience, including the attendant sensations, emotions, thoughts, and actions. And if it is not able to fit into an existing schema, the memory cannot be cognitively assessed, represented in memory, and integrated into the personal narrative or life story of an individual (van der Kolk & van der Hart, 1989, 1991). The dissociated memory then remains split off and unconnected in an "utterly incompatible" world removed from a continuous sense of time (van der Kolk & van der Hart, 1991, p. 448). In this world, the memory may be vivid and fixed, while in normal conscious awareness, it may remain inaccessible (Janet, 1892; van der Kolk et al., 1989; van der Kolk & van der Hart, 1989, 1991).

Horowitz (1991) further articulates the process of dissociation in relation to schemas, noting that

> the "I" designation, usually added to information about one's own mental or bodily experiences, may be set aside. This dissociation of self may reduce emotional reactivity. Intolerable horror or other anguish is avoided by a kind of "not me" rather than "me" designation of perceptions and memories. The dissociation may also occur because the traumatic event is so discordant with previously established schemas. (p. 27)

Particularly for the child whose developing and fragile schemas may be shattered by traumatic information, dissociation may provide an adaptive route to avoidance of decompensation or psychosis. The use of dissociative defenses may result specifically in differential assimilation of new information into discrete meaning networks separated by dissociative barriers or alterations in conscious awareness. Thus cognitive schemas may become segregated, isolating memories into discrete and possibly mutually exclusive dissociative states, or they may be partially or completely severed with various components of the traumatic experience attached to various fragments of the schema. Whichever occurs, defective (i.e., circumscribed and representationally limited) schemas may be the result of dissociative processing.

Summary: Schemas, Trauma, and Memory

Most often, traumatic experience directly threatens existing schemas, needs, and assumptions. With the bulk of everyday experience, new information is automatically assimilated into existing schemas, while gradual and appropriate accommodations of schemas are made to adjust to new learning and current realities. These processes, however, are disrupted by trauma. Assimilation is, in most cases, not immediately possible, as existing schemas provide no frame for understanding the anomaly of the traumatic experience. Accommodation of the schemas to the trauma threaten loss of basic assumptions and needs regarding safety and stability of self in the world. Therefore the trauma may remain unintegrated, at least for a time. Optimally the biphasic pattern of intrusion and denial will titrate assimilation and accommodation such that the trauma is gradually and safely integrated, leaving schemas appropriately adjusted and memories more or less transformed to palatable forms compatible with basic assumptions and understanding (Erdelyi, 1990; Horowitz, 1991). However, this outcome may be circumvented if the trauma is too threatening or the emotion too intense, leaving the experience unintegrated into schematic memory and unrepresented in a form that is meaningful and accessible to conscious awareness. This may result in a loss of the memory, perhaps to a repressed unconscious. Or the memory may be split off through dissociative processes. If the memory is dissociated, it may be unavailable to consciousness while retaining a particular vividness and detail often lost when individual memories are absorbed into the larger meaning matrix of schemas (Barclay, 1986; van der Kolk & van der Hart, 1989). If repressed, such a memory may be fragmented and fused with other unconscious content.

In integrating schema theory as motivation for repression or dissociation, the specific cognitive mechanisms of this motivated forgetting are still open for exploration. What are the effects of trauma and its interaction with schemas on encoding, storage, or retrieval of memories? What are the developmental influences on the nature of encoding and later retrieval? How do these processes affect a continuous sense of narrative? And is the nature of this narrative constructive or historically accurate? These questions are addressed in the following chapters.

T · H · R · E · E

Cognitive Processes
in Trauma and Memory

Clinicians working with both child and adult victims of trauma
have reported a wide variety of memory attributes ranging from
eidetic vividness to complete absences of conscious memory.
Clinical theory has addressed these varying presentations of
memory in terms of repression and dissociation, with more
recent integrative thinking incorporating schema theory as well.
However, these concepts neither adequately address the mechanisms underlying traumatic memory, nor fully explain the wide
range of memory attributes described in clinical populations. In
elucidating these phenomena, integrating clinical theories with
cognitive research and theory may enhance the ability of both
clinicians and cognitive scientists to understand memory for
early trauma.

Although memories, traumatic and otherwise, are represented in various modalities (verbal, affective, motoric, etc.), it is
most often assumed that verbal representation is necessary for
the achievement of full conscious awareness and recall. When
conscious awareness and recall are not possible, thus when
memory is impaired, the disruption in the processing of verbal
representation may involve interactions between the dynamic

sequelae of trauma (such as terror or helplessness) and various memory processes including encoding, storage, and retrieval. Further, to understand such mechanisms relative to the memory functioning of an adult who has experienced childhood trauma, it first is necessary to understand normative memory development and functioning.

Normal Memory in Children: Research Findings

A growing body of empirical literature addresses normative memory functioning in infants and young children. This literature is shifting from consideration of discontinuities in the development of memory to support for the idea that memory development is a continuous process. Specifically, long-held theoretical positions suggested that, in very young children, developing memory systems are not initially functional, leaving only chaotic traces and unconnected fragments with no contextual or temporal organization (e.g., Piaget, 1969). Abrupt developmental shifts have been proposed to explain the transition from an ineffective memory system to a mature, effective memory functioning. A variety of mechanisms ranging from repression to neurology have been offered for this developmental dysfunction; however, little controlled research has supported such claims.

The increasingly held opinion, in fact, is that these theories are incorrect, as research repeatedly demonstrates sophisticated memory abilities in infants and children who appear capable of organizing, sequencing, and retaining memories from the earliest months of life. For example, several studies of very young infants and preschool children demonstrating continuity in memory functioning found organized and accurate behavioral and/or verbal memories for real-life events. These memories were maintained even over long-term retention intervals, and they manifested evidence of temporal and spatial sensitivity, discrimination of novel elements, conceptual ability, possible generalization and analogical application, associative encoding and reactivation of seemingly forgotten experiences, and resistance to suggestion or distortion of an event's central essence. Further, studies suggest a basic continuity in the nature of infant and adult memory processes, and they show long-term retention in children at ages prior to the offset of childhood amnesia, calling into question certain theories of childhood amnesia relative to developmental discontinuity (e.g., Bauer, 1995; Bauer, Hertsgaard, & Dow, 1994; Bauer & Mandler, 1990; Eth, 1988; Farrar & Goodman, 1990; Fivush & Hamond, 1990; Goodman, Rudy, Bottoms, & Aman, 1990; Howe & Courage, 1993; Howe, O'Sullivan, & Marche, 1992; Hudson, 1990; Liwag & Stein, 1995; Meltzoff, 1995; Nelson, 1988, 1990; Nurcombe, 1986; Ornstein, Gordon, & Baker-Ward, 1992; Rovee-Collier & Shyi, 1992; Sheffield & Hudson, 1994; Toglia, Ross, Ceci, & Hembrooke, 1992).

Memory distortions or errors noted in these studies of young children's memories include confusion of details over repeated events, inconsistencies over recall trials due to nature of cues provided, errors of omission, misunderstandings of language use due to nascent lingual abilities, and forgetting or reordering specific objects in a sequence. In almost all of these studies, the distortions found in the memories left the essence intact and were related primarily to verbal memory. Even with often successful attempts to inculcate misinformation, children's memories for real events (queried by both free recall and misleading, suggestive questioning) most often yielded accuracy for essence, particularly when attempts were made to insert abuse or trauma-related misinformation (Goodman et al., 1990; Goodman, Hirschman, Hepps, & Rudy, 1991; Ornstein et al., 1992).

However, in spite of these most often very robust findings demonstrating well-developed memory capacities in young children, much debate exists over whether such studies demonstrate implicit (i.e., procedural) memories or explicit (i.e., episodic) memories. This debate is focused on the idea that conscious, verbally mediated awareness is a prerequisite for defining a memory as explicit. Thus infants cannot possibly be "remembering" as such. In response to this assumption, Howe and Courage (1993) note that "because no one would argue that memory operates in an exclusively conscious or verbal mode, especially early in life, infantile amnesia may be a chimera, an epiphenomenon rather than a phenomenon" (p. 316). Moreover, disagreement exists as to whether there are even such multiple memory systems, rather than a more complex, flexibly operating single memory system (Nelson, 1994).

Although many prefer a precise definition of memory specified by clear, conscious, episodic recall, here we are interested in myriad ways of expressing memory for early events. Where it is possible to denote distinctions between various memory functions (or systems), an attempt will be made to do so. However, this discussion will explore early memory in all of its understood and demonstrated manifestations. A range of such manifestations can be seen in memories for childhood trauma.

Representations of Trauma in Memory: Research Findings

Although much literature, empirical and theoretical, addresses the effects of trauma on memory, few studies offer full, systematic, descriptive exploration of this phenomenon beyond clinical case studies and anecdotal information. Since trauma cannot ethically be reproduced in the laboratory, ecologically valid research on the nature of trauma and memory necessarily has involved observational and phenomenological studies of survivors in field studies.

Janet was one of the first to describe the clinical manifestations of traumatic memory. From systematic observations of
more than 5,000 patients, he concluded that traumatic memory
has all-or-none, inflexible, invariable, and nonsocial (or autistic)
components. He also noted that traumatic memory is decontextualized in that a meaningful (often verbally encoded) context
is absent. Further the time sense and historical placement of
traumatic memory is disrupted (van der Kolk & van der Hart,
1991).

Harvey and Herman (1994) report clinical cases charac-
terizing three general patterns of traumatic remembrance. First
is continuous and complete recall coupled with delayed understanding of these experiences, as in a child who is sexually abused
but has too little knowledge of normative experience to attrib-
ute traumatic meaning to the event. Second is partial amnesia
for components of the traumatic event, coupled with some
delayed recall and delayed understanding, as in an adult who has
a few distinct memories but later recalls additional memories,
increasing the impact of the events. And finally these authors
note a pattern of delayed recall following complete amnesia for
the events. In regard to these patterns, Harvey and Herman
(1994) characterize a typical adult survivor of early trauma as

> a person who arrives at adulthood with some, but not all,
> memories of the abuse intact, and who at some point in
> time begins to confront and rethink the past, blending new
> memories with earlier ones, new assessments with alterna-
> tive ones, gradually constructing a meaningful and largely
> verifiable personal history: a history that is patently "true"
> though never complete and never wholly accurate in all
> detail. (p. 303)

Lenore Terr (1983, 1988, 1990, 1991) has conducted extensive field studies of survivors of trauma. Terr has written much
about a longitudinal study of 25 school children (ages 5 to 14)

who, with their schoolbus driver, were kidnapped, buried alive, and left to die (Terr, 1983, 1988). All eventually escaped, and at assessments conducted at 1 year and 4 to 5 years after the incident, she found that most of these children retained clear, detailed verbal memories, in spite of active attempts to suppress or avoid thinking about the event. In addition, she also observed very specific behavioral memories (e.g., play, fears, motoric reenactments) but noted a lack of affective memory in many of her subjects. She noted that the fullness of their memories was not dependent on any parental intervention or repetition in discussing or processing the event and that any forgetting that had occurred concerned events following the kidnapping and not the kidnapping itself. Further, over the 4- to 5-year interval, she found little to no modification of the original memories, noting that the memories for these children had remained vivid, detailed, and "intensely alive" (1990, p. 174). The degree to which such traumatic memories remain intact may be attributable to the fact that the survivors tend to suppress thought and discussion concerning the traumatic events, leaving the memories more or less unrehearsed and, thus, with little of the attendant modification or interference (Terr, 1994).

In another retrospective study, Terr (1988, 1990) reviewed charts and extensive notes she had taken on 20 children she had seen for trauma consultation or treatment. The children's ages ranged from 6 months to 4 years at the time of the trauma, and her evaluations took place an average of 4 years after the traumas. She found that, regardless of age, most of her subjects had exhibited some form of memory for the trauma, with impairment more often seen with repeated traumas. The representations of trauma in memory were encoded in verbal, behavioral, or motoric (play, gestures), positional/postural or spatial, sensory (smells, sounds), affective (fears), physiological (tingling in a specific spot, choking), or personality-based (specific, repetitive interpersonal responses) modalities. Terr's observation was that across modalities, and regardless of age of trauma, the memories were highly accurate and specific to the traumatic event, even in nonconscious (i.e., nonverbal) modalities (1988). She acknowledged that while her access to detailed and verified documentation of the traumas in these children enabled her to trace the specificity and accuracy of the responses, a retrospective interpretation of nonverbal memories without such documentation would be difficult (Terr, 1988). However, in the absence of such documentation, Terr (1994) does offer one criterion for interpreting the validity and meaning of such symptoms. She suggests that nonverbal symptomatic behaviors following trauma may be a part of the behavioral repertoire for a lifetime, often taking on the characteristic of "lifelong motifs" (p. 56). The sudden appearance of nonverbal reenactments following the recovery of traumatic memory may lead one to consider the veracity of the memory or the dynamic meaning of such a presentation.

When considering the differences in vivid memories versus fragmented or absent memories, Terr (1990, 1991) concluded that memories (i.e., verbal and other modalities) for single traumatic experiences remain more or less intact with some distortion, while memories (primarily verbal) for repeated traumas manifest significant impairment. She theoretically supported this finding by positing that sudden, unexpected events may overwhelm cognitive and emotional defenses, focusing attention and memory. However, chronic trauma occurring over repeated episodes may stimulate defensive operations (such as denial, splitting, self-anesthesia, and dissociation) that serve to block from full consciousness expected traumatic realities, thus preserving the developing self (Terr, 1990, 1994). These defenses then may disrupt attentional, encoding, storage, or retrieval processes, resulting in full or partial loss of traumatic memories. Further, chronic trauma may be subject to secrecy or distortion by others involved in its chronicity, as in sexual abuse, also contributing to memory impairment (Enns, McNeilly, Corkery, & Gilbert, 1995; Terr, 1990).

Terr has found, however, that even with memory losses, the remaining or recovered *essence* of traumatic memory is generally intact, accurate, and long-lasting. She concluded from her research that at any age, at least in visual and/or sensory modalities, impressions of trauma are "burned-in" (1988, p. 103). In a similar study with adults, Herman (1992), too, noted a predominance of accurate imagery and bodily sensation (often in the absence of verbal narrative). Pynoos and Nader (1989) studied children who were involved in a school playground shooting spree and also noted basically intact visual and verbal memories.

In spite of high degrees of accuracy, memory impairments do, of course, occur. These impairments include distortions, errors, and memory losses. In a laboratory analogue study examining the effects of stress on memory, Christianson and Nilsson (1984) found amnesia for items associated with traumatic events. In a clinical sample by Herman and Schatzow (1987), 64% of subjects with trauma histories showed some memory impairment or loss, with 28% showing severe memory loss, with greater memory loss correlating with greater severity of violence and younger age of victim. The memories that were available did, however, tend to be accurate, as 74% of the sample corroborated their memories with external verification. In similar studies, Briere and Conte (1993) found that almost 60% of their subjects had some amnesia for early childhood abuse, and Williams (1994a, 1994b) found that 38% of women with documented early traumas did not report remembering these traumas as adults. In this study, an additional 16% reported forgetting the trauma at some point in life, while remembering with accuracy at the time of the interview. Williams (1994a) concluded that these results demonstrated forgetting significantly beyond the rate predicted by childhood amnesia. Although these studies have been criticized for methodological or interpretive flaws, their authors defend the support demonstrated for the possibility that early trauma can be, and often is, inaccessible to adult memory.

In addition to amnesias, however, memory impairment often includes errors and distortions. Such impairments in Terr's subjects usually manifested as errors in time sense (duration, sequence, etc.), modality transfer (an event originally subject to auditory encoding transfers to a visual image as the individual "sees" what has occurred), subtraction (suppressed affect), addition of details, or condensation (Terr, 1988, 1990). Pynoos and Nader (1989) observed no errors in sequencing or duration but did observe distortions that were spatially focused. In their sample, children in close proximity to a violent event minimized the degree of life threat, while children further away and thus less threatened perceived increased life threat on recall.

Finally, others have observed that memory impairment after trauma seems to be centered on episodic (or explicit) memory, whereas semantic (or implicit) memory resulting from the traumatic event remains intact and accurate. This observation is demonstrated by clients with clear, repetitive memories evidenced in nonverbal modalities (behaviors, fears, interpersonal sequences) that may be nonconscious or, if conscious, without obvious meaning or awareness of the original learning context (Kihlstrom & Hoyt, 1990; Spiegel et al., 1993). Other studies have demonstrated similar profiles of traumatic memory in children or in adults who experienced childhood trauma (Ewin, 1994; Freud, 1892b, 1896; Herman, 1992; Herman & Schatzow, 1987; Howe & Courage, 1993; Levis, 1990; Loftus, 1994).

There is debate over the nature of "traumatic memory" per se relative to its existence as a unique memory process distinct from "normal memory." Nonetheless, there are suggestions that trauma may have a significant impact on memory functioning due to frequently complicating factors including secrecy; shame and guilt; negative responses of others; high arousal, terror, and helplessness; inability to escape; and the often devastating meaning of trauma in one's life (Enns et al., 1995; Williams, 1994b).

Normal Memory Functioning, Childhood Amnesia, and Trauma

If childhood memory systems are so continuous and well-functioning, what, then, explains forgetting, motivated or otherwise? Several hypotheses are offered. In considering the variation in the attributes of traumatic memories, the mechanisms underlying such memories will be examined relative to normative functioning of memory in children, and these mechanisms will be considered relative to the memory impairments often seen in trauma. Although memory for early trauma may be disrupted by any of the dynamic, defensive, or cognitive factors discussed in previous chapters, much attention has been directed specifically toward the phenomenon of childhood amnesia as a potential explanation for impairment of memory for early traumas.

Freud and other early clinicians and theorists noted that most adults have little to no memory for events occurring prior to the age of 5 years. Historically, descriptions of childhood amnesia arose from anecdotal, clinical, and subjective accounts of difficulties in recall for early events (Freud, 1917; Piaget, 1962; Waldvogel, 1948). More recently, however, retrospective memory studies have documented adults' inability to remember early experiences by applying linear retention functions based on normal forgetting rates and observing significant, discontinuous drops at the age period thought to mark childhood amnesia (Fitzgerald, 1990; Wetzler & Sweeney, 1986).

Some theoretical explanations for childhood amnesia assume the fundamental developmental discontinuity discussed earlier, positing early childhood cognitive processing to be very dissimilar in both form and function to adult cognition. Such discontinuities have been thought to lead to the inability to appropriately encode or store early memories, and, by extension, to the inability to remember early traumatic experiences. Another body of thought, again perhaps more empirically based, challenges the assumption of developmental discontinuity, suggesting that, in fact, memory development exists on a continuum with early memory functioning in a fashion that is more similar than dissimilar to adult memory, with specific structural and functional systems in place at very early ages. Thus the retention of early memory is less dependent on qualitative developmental shifts than on gradual maturation as well as on specific factors related to encoding, storage, rehearsal, and retrieval context. Several theories representing both perspectives for understanding childhood amnesia will be briefly considered.

EARLY THEORIES

Freud attributed childhood amnesia to the repression of unacceptable infantile wishes involving sexual and aggressive themes (Freud, 1896, 1917). Piaget (1962) and others attributed childhood amnesia to factors involving qualitative developmental shifts in cognitive capacities, such as the progression from sensorimotor to formal operational thought. Schachtel (1947, 1959) suggested that a child's basic experience of the world is so unique in its intensity and lack of cognitive structure that adulthood renders one unable to return to such experience. A child experiences and assimilates new experience before the development of language and schemas, leaving such experience unable to be retained or retrieved in meaningful ways. Without adult schematic representation, childhood experience has "no suitable vessels (schemata) for its preservation" (Schachtel, 1959, p. 298). Due to myriad developmental shifts, Schachtel (1947, 1959) even suggested that childhood and adult memory systems are "mutually alien" (1959, p. 306). Thus from this viewpoint, both everyday memories and traumatic memories of childhood are unintelligible and inassimilable to adult cognition. If fragments are available or recovered, they will exist only in a vivid, strange, and fragmented form, as they have been isolated and unable to form associations with current schemas and autobiographical memories (Fitzgerald, 1990; Parkin, 1987; Schachtel, 1959; Waldvogel, 1948). Other theories of developmental discontinuities contributing to child–adult memory incompatibility include shifts in neurophysiology (discussed in the next chapter) and the balance or salience of receptor systems associated with cognitive development (e.g., from childhood "near-receptor" dominance [smell, touch] to adulthood "far-receptor" dominance [vision, hearing]) (White & Pillemer, 1979).

DUAL MEMORY SYSTEMS

Pillemer and White (1989) have proposed an early primitive memory system qualitatively different from a later autobiographical system. Specifically, the early system contains only fragmentary information and generalized knowledge evoked by specific cues and primarily expressed in behavioral rather than verbal modalities. The second system, emerging later in development, allows temporally and contextually based personal memories that can be accessed on demand and communicated verbally. The immaturity or absence of this latter, socially accessible, system may explain childhood amnesia.

Assuming at least dual memory systems, some research supports the idea that young children show evidence only of procedural or "habit" learning, with episodic (and autobiographical) memory appearing later in development. This theory defines "memory" per se as conscious, episodically organized, and most often verbally mediated. Thus from this position, it appears that children lack the capacity for memory as defined and are capable only of generalized learning that is not accessible to conscious, episodic recall. As such, young children may encode information that can be organized and later utilized, most often in nonverbal form, but they cannot retain memories of an episodic nature (e.g., McDonough & Mandler, 1994). Although a body of research interprets findings as demonstrating episodic recall in preverbal children, little evidence exists to confirm that these memories are of a specific nature involving memory of the actual learning event (Fivush, 1994a; Pillemer & White, 1989). In fact, without a clear demonstration of verbal organization and mediation, no current paradigm can unequivocally demonstrate episodic recall. Although many cognitive scientists have developed paradigms producing results that cannot be attributed to conditioned learning or expression of generalized memory, a gap remains between these certainties and the demonstration of episodic recall. Thus this theory suggests that while adults do retain procedural and semantic knowledge gained throughout development, memories of an episodic nature (such as memories for specific traumatic events early in life) may be unavailable to voluntary recall.

FUZZY TRACE THEORY

Fuzzy trace theory involves the integrity and detail of memory traces relative to encoding, storage, and retrieval. In general this theory considers the differential levels of trace detail on a continuum from very detailed, exact, verbatim traces to abstract or gist-like (i.e., fuzzy) traces. A single memory, encoded through a process of pattern recognition (i.e., shape, contour, size, etc.) followed by interpretive analysis (i.e., attaching meaning, forming semantic associations, assigning emotional valence, etc.), may be redundantly encoded on both ends of this verbatim-to-fuzzy continuum at once, with retrieval preference given to the fuzzy or gist-like trace. Thus, information at one level of abstractness (i.e., fuzzy traces) may be retrieved, while at other levels (i.e., verbatim) the traces are unavailable for immediate recall. This pattern may be related to the tendency for verbatim traces to necessitate greater complexity of cognitive processing and to disintegrate at faster rates, while fuzzy traces require less complex processing, are retained for longer periods, and appear more resistant to suggestion or modification from competing experiences (Ceci & Bruck, 1993; Leichtman & Ceci, 1993; Reyna, 1992).

In a young child, the conceptual ability needed to transform perceptual–motor experiences into abstract propositional representations (i.e., interpretive gist-like traces) may require considerable development. And the fuzzy traces that do exist, especially in preverbal children, may lend themselves less easily to intentional, socially induced recall than to nonverbal expression. Further, the profusion of traces at the verbatim end of the continuum are likely inadequately encoded due to the immaturity of the young child's lingual and representational abilities, and such memories are, in general, subject to more rapid decay. As a result, memories encoded prior to the enhanced ability for extracting and conceptualizing gist may appear inaccessible to conscious, verbal recall (Leichtman & Ceci, 1993; Reyna, 1992). Thus trauma that occurs very early in life, may tend toward verbatim rather than gist encoding, leaving the traumatic experience largely uninterpreted and the memory traces less likely to be given retrieval preference. Further, these early verbatim traces should decay more rapidly, rendering them unavailable for retrieval in adulthood.

LANGUAGE ACQUISITION

Another related developmental marker potentially significant in childhood memory is the acquisition of language. Language serves a function in cognitive representation as well as social communication, both of which may have an impact on memory functioning. Specifically, the acquisition of language creates an ability for verbal encoding with its attendant organization and

elaborative complexity, enhancing the capacity to verbally mediate, and thus better comprehend, experiences in the world. In
other words, lingual ability allows interpretation and assignment
of meaning. At least for some kinds of early trauma, without
comprehension of social norms and boundaries, the preverbal
child may not understand (or encode) an event as traumatic
(Loftus, Garry, & Feldman, 1994). Therefore the onset of language may introduce a significant cognitive maturation that
allows for greater consolidation and elaboration in memorial
systems due, in part, to enhanced ability to organize experience
in a narrative form (Ceci & Bruck, 1993; Fivush, Haden, & Adam,
1995; Goodman, Quas, Batterman-Faunce, Riddlesberger, &
Kuhn, 1994; Nelson, 1993; Pillemer & White, 1989).

The shift in language ability may also render early nonverbal
memory (particularly involving episodic or event memory) less
accessible to consciousness if, in fact, these memories ever even
achieved that status. Specifically, a theory of encoding specificity
suggests that the modality of initial encoding may be unlikely to
translate or transfer to another modality. For example, the original
encoding of a preverbal child who behaviorally reenacts a traumatic event is likely to be nonverbal (e.g., image-based); thus, the
original encoding for this event is unlikely to transfer to a verbal
modality that might allow later verbal mediation and conscious
remembrance of the early event (Sugar, 1992). This theory, while
not disconfirmed to any significant extent empirically, has been
challenged by several striking anecdotal accounts demonstrating
modality transfer from preverbal to verbal mediation of traumatic
memories (e.g., see Boyer, Barron, & Farrar, 1994; Hewitt, 1994;
McDonough & Mandler, 1994; Myers, Perris, & Speaker, 1994).
Further, a child with nascent lingual abilities may need adult
structuring or scaffolding to capture early experience through
verbal description. If a traumatized child is not supported in
understanding and organizing his or her experience in this way,
later memorability may be impaired.

Related to this need for adult mediation, a second function of language arises. Specifically, as young children gain increasing language facility, they learn through interactions with significant adults that language serves a social communicative function that includes the remembrance and retelling of memories for past events. Social exchange demands the ability to produce ideas in an organized symbolic mode that denotes time, space, and causation (White & Pillemer, 1979).

Serving functions for both cultural transmission and interpersonal exchange, this use of language also may mediate memory ability and, indeed, has been empirically and theoretically supported as a basis for the development of the autobiographical memory system (Tessler & Nelson, 1994). Nelson (1994) notes that "human lives take root in social and symbolic worlds in which the significance of events is determined by one's place and role in those events, thus establishing their memorability" (p. 474). As such, the onset of language, autobiographical memory, and narrative capabilities allows the sharing of experiences in ways that contribute to an understanding of their significance relative to the social milieu and one's own selfhood (Barclay, 1994; Howe & Courage, 1993; Hudson, 1990; Nelson, 1988, 1990, 1993, 1994; Tessler & Nelson, 1994).

Specifically, the very young child who is incapable of using verbal language in interpersonal exchanges has little, if any, understanding of the social value of remembering. This child neither knows "how" to remember or "why" such an activity may be important beyond an involuntary retention of procedural knowledge necessary for survival. As a child acquires language, however, adults "scaffold" experience for the child, supporting comprehension as well as marking which aspects are important for memory. Subsequent rehearsal of shared experiences reinforces these functions as well as models for the developing child retrieval strategies for later internalization (Boyer et al., 1994).

This idea is consistent with a Vygotskian perspective suggesting that skills develop first in social interaction, only later to be internalized by the developing child. Studies of conversation between primary caregivers and their children have documented this process of learning "how" and "why" to remember and emphasizing the value of skills for the exchange of such information (Boyer et al., 1994; Fivush, 1991; Fivush et al., 1995; Hudson, 1993; Mandler, 1990; Nelson, 1993, 1994; Pillemer & White, 1989). Thus develops a "performance system that produces symbols that can be read by others who will then understand what the child knows or remembers" (White & Pillemer, 1979, p. 62). However, given the status of most forms of trauma as socially unacceptable and undesirable for cultural transmission, the social value in remembering and communicating details of traumatic experiences is diminished. Further, if the scaffolding provided by adults is intentionally distorted (e.g., a perpetrator applies distorted meaning to an abuse episode, or a protective parent reframes a traumatic event as other than traumatic), then memory may also be impaired.

SELF-DEVELOPMENT

Incorporating many of the above ideas, a final theory of childhood amnesia involves the development of self in the growing child. Although the very concept of "self" has eluded clear and precise definition, it has been operationalized variably in research exploring early physical self-recognition, manifestations of self-consciousness, reflexive language use, pronoun use, awareness of agency, and other components that are thought to reflect the development of a coherent self-structure in the child (Howe & Courage, 1993).

This theory suggests that the development of a self is a necessary prerequisite to the development of an autobiographical memory system involving memories for personally meaningful events situated in context and time. It is thought that a self-structure provides a sort of internal scaffolding through which such memories can cohere and elaborate (Howe, Courage, & Peterson, 1994). In turn, such memories can provide a means for "understanding and representing the self as continuous in time" (Fivush et al., 1995, p. 34). In fact, Howe and Courage (1993) note that "infantile amnesia devolves as knowledge of the self evolves and that the emergence of the infant's sense of self is the fundamental cornerstone in the development of autobiographical memory" (p. 306). Similarly, Nelson (1993), in discussing self-development and memory, suggests that "the onset of autobiographical memory is simply the inverse of infantile amnesia" (p. 8).

Some research has demonstrated that conceptions of self begin to emerge around the time of early language acquisition. These developmental milestones may interact in that language provides the ability for developing a narrative of one's life, thus contributing to the development of self and autobiographical memory; likewise, the development of self may provide a focus around which language can be used to organize memories and to create such a narrative (Howe & Courage, 1993; Fivush et al., 1995; Nelson, 1993; Neisser, 1994). With early trauma, the lack of self-development may render the events less meaningful as well as less memorable, as no sufficient autobiographical memory system yet exists to retain such memories. Further, early trauma can, itself, interfere with the process of self-development, creating a negative feedback loop of disruption in self- and memory functioning (similar to such processes as articulated in Chapter 2).

Cognitive Mechanisms
and Unavailability of Early Memories

In addition to these more elaborated theories of childhood amnesia, other considerations of the inaccessibility of early traumatic material to memory involve specific cognitive mechanisms that operate in both "normal" and traumatic memory processing, if, in fact, such a distinction can be made. In a simplistic structure breaking memory down into processes of encoding, storage, and retrieval, several factors will be explored.

ENCODING

A wealth of studies focus on encoding processes in demonstrating that young children in the process of laying down schemas for comprehension and prediction of the world initially attend to and encode general, representative, or typical aspects of events and attend less, if at all, to novel aspects. This process merges repeated or similar experiences into general schemas at the cost of detail for specific episodes and memory for novel episodes (e.g., Bauer, 1995; Hudson, 1986, 1993). Thus recall of events occurring in this developmental stage might capture the essence while distorting detail in the direction of schematic prediction and ignoring anomalies.

Once schemas are established and related feature and pattern detection more or less automatic, schemas shape which features in an event are attended to, encoded, and understood, biasing attentional processes toward schema-confirming information, particularly for young children who have been shown to be more reliant on schemas for processing experience and memories (Barclay, 1986; Ceci & Bruck, 1993; Hudson, 1986, 1993; Mandler, 1983). In fact, the attributes of individualized schemas may be responsible, in part, for individual differences in traumatic memory (Bonanno, 1990b). Developed schemas also can be used to detect anomalies or novelties that then are noticed as distinct (relative to the schemas) and retained in a separate, autobiographical memory system linked to, but not embedded within, the appropriate schema. Trauma, most often an anomalous experience, is subject to this process; however, if chronically repeated, details may be fused or inaccessible, as they may be absorbed in a larger, trauma-based schema (Bartlett, 1932; Farrar & Goodman, 1990; Fivush et al., 1995; Howe & Courage, 1993; Hudson, 1986, 1993; Mandler, 1990; Murray, 1988; Neisser, 1986, 1988, 1990; Nelson, 1994; Schachtel, 1959; Singer & Salovey, 1991). In other terms, the young child may initially develop semantic memory processes, providing basic schemas containing knowledge about the world (even trauma-based knowledge), and only later develop episodic memory processes capable of encoding and retaining distinct personal memories. However, the development of these systems is not mutually exclusive (Fitzgerald, 1990; Loftus, 1979; Nurcombe, 1986; Schachtel, 1959; Tulving, 1984, 1985; White & Pillemer, 1979).

This developmental process ensures the adaptive allocation of early resources to the organization of experience. However, the nature of this developmental sequence at any stage may be preempted in traumatic, life-threatening situations during which the obvious adaptive stance would direct focal attention to the specific precipitating event (Farrar & Goodman, 1990; Fitzgerald, 1990; Fivush & Hamond, 1990; Hudson, 1990; Howe & Courage, 1993; Nelson, 1988; Ratner, Smith, & Padgett, 1990; Rovee-Collier & Shyi, 1992).

Although debate exists concerning the facilitative or inhibitory effects of traumatic stress on such processes, Neisser (1990) suggests that perhaps such effects are mediated by novelty (which may determine the degree of differentiation and complexity of an experience) as well as by degree of involvement (participant or observer). The more novel the experience, as suggested previously, and the higher the degree of personal involvement or participation, the better the event is remembered. Goodman and colleagues (1990) studied somewhat novel situations (doctor visits requiring inoculations) and found that children 3 to 6 years old demonstrating high stress responses recalled more of the experience, were less suggestible to misleading information, and provided details that were completely accurate. However, Howe and colleagues (1994) found no effects of stress on long-term retention in a sample of young children receiving emergency room treatment. In a similar study, only a high degree of stress or emotional arousal had effects on memory, facilitating both accuracy and accessibility of memories (Goodman et al., 1991). Others have found enhanced accuracy for certain details of a stressful situation and decreased accuracy for others. Specifically, it may be that to enhance survival, stress narrows attentional processes (i.e., attentional selectivity) toward encoding only of gist and associated central details at the expense of peripheral details; or it may be that they are differentially elaborated (Christianson & Loftus, 1990, 1991; Burke, Heuer, & Reisberg, 1992; Christianson & Nilsson, 1989). Or, as Ceci and Bruck (1993) suggest, stress at encoding could enhance storage, whereas stress at retrieval could impair access to contents of storage.

Further clarifying the effects of trauma on encoding and early memory, Christianson and Nilsson (1989) suggest that in trauma, arousal level is related to the degree to which coping activities and perseverative tendencies are directed toward critical aspects of the event. They posit a "cue-utilization theory" that suggests an inverted-U-shaped relationship between arousal and attention to cues such that certain levels of arousal result in decreased ability for parallel processing due to a demand for resources by focused attention and physiological responses (1989, p. 297). The resulting restriction in elaboration may limit cues available to aid retrieval later.

Similarly, attentional processes related to traumatic arousal may be focused or narrowed in the sense of "motivated non-learning" wherein thought-stopping or avoidance begins as a conscious process and becomes, through practice, automatic (Bower, 1990, p. 219). Especially in repeated traumas, this means that a dissociative-like process occurs that originally is intentional and, through use, becomes automatic, interfering with encoding processes (Kihlstrom & Hoyt, 1990). Thus initial registration, categorization, and elaborative processing are restricted, probably in order to titrate negative emotion.

Other theorists consider the effects of modality utilized to encode incoming stimuli. Extensive developmental research, building on the theories of Piaget (1970), has identified three primary modes of representation in memory: enactive or motoric, involving motor activity; iconic or imagistic, incorporating sensory input; and symbolic or conceptual (or verbal), utilizing higher levels of reasoning, language, abstraction, and organization (Bruner, 1964, cited in Bonanno, 1990a, 1990b; Horowitz, 1988, 1992; Mandler, 1983; van der Kolk & van der Hart, 1991). Of these three modes of representation, it is generally assumed that conceptual (i.e., verbal) representation is necessary for full conscious awareness (Greenberg & van der Kolk, 1987). Particularly in trauma, the emotional intensity may result in "speechless terror" outside comprehensible human experience, precluding assimilation on a symbolic/conceptual or verbal level, and leaving encoding processes to occur in enactive and iconic modalities, leaving the memory for the event unavailable for conscious, verbal recall (Erdelyi & Goldberg, 1979; Pillemer & White, 1989; van der Kolk & van der Hart, 1991, p. 443). Further, a preverbal child will possess neither the lingual ability nor the comprehension of meaning, leaving limited possibilities for later recall on a conceptual level. Thus memories may take nonlinguistic forms (motoric enactments, images, sensory impressions), making later conscious comprehension difficult (Hudson, 1993). Or if memories are encoded on all three levels, a defensive cleavage may preempt the normal conscious flow between them, rendering one or more of the modalities inhibited, as in dissociative processes (Horowitz, 1988; Bonanno, 1990a).

A more detailed variation on this model specifies a parallel distributed processing network in which memories are encoded and stored in dynamic networks (much like neuronal networks). These networks comprise many interconnected computing units that form patterns of activation through varying configurations of excitation or inhibition. Activation in the network spreads by propagating along connections between units (Spiegel, 1990; Stinson & Palmer, 1991). In this model, a memory can be thought of as a "distributed representation" encoded as a network defined by a specific pattern of activation over multiple units, each of which code specific details (i.e., "microfeatures") of an object or event (Stinson & Palmer, 1991, p. 349). The successful encoding of memories requires integration of the network, possibly dependent on integration of a unified self-structure or schema. In the absence of such integration, caused perhaps by traumatic experience, components of memories may be encoded in a dissociated manner, isolating various representational fragments and rendering them less likely to be retrieved (Bonanno, 1990a; McNally, 1993; Stinson & Palmer, 1991).

STORAGE OR RETENTION

Other theorists have empirically supported the hypothesis that impairment of childhood memories is due to storage failure. The "trace-integrity model" (which actually applies to both storage and recall) suggests that "both forgetting and reminiscence are represented along a single (trace integrity) continuum in which the critical component is variation in the 'strength' of the bonds that unite features" of a memory and associations to that memory (Howe, Kelland, Bryant-Brown, & Clark, 1992, p. 62; McNally, 1993; Pezdek & Roe, 1994, 1995; Toglia et al., 1992).

Forgetting is, in part, due to decreases in the strength of these associative bonds over time. The rapidity with which these traces decay is dependent upon several factors including encoding elaboration, rehearsal, interference, and encoding specificity

(Toglia et al., 1992). With increased decay of trace strength come a decreased ability to discriminate distinct traces from background noise of other traces as well as a decreased number of associative links to these traces (Howe et al., 1992). Further, the loose integration of weak traces may allow intrusion and incorporation of other information that may coexist with or even overwrite the original trace (Ceci & Bruck, 1993).

If not erased, a disintegrated trace can, however, be rebuilt (or "redintegrated") thus reactivating the memory trace (Howe et al., 1992, p. 63; Sheffield & Hudson, 1994; Toglia et al., 1992) through initiation of rehearsal (e.g., in the form of concentrated thinking) resulting in memory recovery that can be plotted on a function much like an inversion of a classic forgetting function (Erdelyi, 1990). However, this process may introduce the possibility for distortion in the inclusion of postevent information (Ceci & Bruck, 1993). It may be that young children are particularly susceptible to such a process, as it is thought that they tend to encode weaker, less elaborated and integrated traces that primarily exist on the more vulnerable verbatim end of the fuzzy-to-verbatim continuum (Ceci & Bruck, 1993; Pezdek & Roe, 1995). The exception to this may be found in frequently rehearsed or repeated experiences that create stronger traces.

This model is similar to the parallel distributed processing model noted above, which also suggests that during storage, perseverative processing involving activation–inhibition exchanges within and between various networks has effects on the strengths or weights of the associative bonds, which in turn determine the strength of the integrated memory (Spiegel, 1990). This model addresses traumatic amnesia: "The fact that content learned may persist despite dense amnesia to the episode in which it was learned can be accounted for by activation of weightings in the net, despite the loss of the weightings associated with the episode itself" (Spiegel, 1990, p. 123). In other words, some sort of dissociative process may separate features of the traumatic episode, leaving some features, such as learned associations, accessible and rendering others inaccessible due to lack of connection to the larger network activation pattern.

The decay in associative bonds (or weightings) may be the result of nonrehearsal. For example, semantic memory seems to remain continuous and intact most likely because it is recalled and utilized, while episodic memories are recalled with less frequency and thus are more subject to decay (Schachtel, 1959).

Further, nonrehearsal of episodic memories may be due to lack of salience or to emotional factors motivating avoidance of the memory (Williams, 1994b; Terr, 1994). This issue is relevant to traumatic memory processing in that avoidance of traumatic emotions such as terror and helplessness may lead to nonrehearsal, decreasing performance of episodic memory. However, event salience may increase rehearsal, at least of certain features of the event, or involuntary rehearsal through nightmares or intrusive imagery may occur, enhancing memory performance (Goodman et al., 1994; Warren & Swartwood, 1992). Individual differences in memory performance may be related to the degree of event salience relative to providing information necessary for future survival versus the degree of threat activated by the intensity of evoked emotions. The rehearsal of selected aspects of the network, and nonrehearsal of others, may be possible through dissociations in the network. Also for emotional reasons, motivated avoidance may cause a memory to be blocked from elaborative processing, limiting the number of associative links to other contents of the memory system (Bonanno, 1990a; Erdelyi, 1990). Or, a traumatized child may selectively and intentionally rehearse certain nonrelevant details of an event (e.g., a child may fixate on shifting patterns of sunlight on a wall during a traumatic event), creating interference with the essence of the traumatic memory.

Further, early rehearsal may be blocked if adults in the child's environment fail to provide the necessary retrieval cues, search strategies, and scaffolding of memorial experience (Fivush & Hamond, 1990). If adults are involved in the trauma, or if they determine that suppressing recall of its occurrence is in the child's best interest, elaboration may be disrupted.

Finally, once in storage, there is speculation that memories can be altered, particularly in high-stress situations. Studies have shown that memories can be supplemented with external information, possibly altered with new associative connections formed with repeated recall, or transformed through suggestion, misleading information, or verbal labels, particularly over the passage of time (Loftus, 1979; Loftus & Christianson, 1989; Loftus & Kaufman, 1992; Loftus & Loftus, 1980). Loftus (1993) cites many examples of inaccuracies in memories of observers of traumatic events. She even cites instances where whole memories have been implanted (e.g., Piaget's "memory" of his own attempted kidnapping as a young child, a story fabricated by his nanny), although some clinicians deny the ability to influence significantly, much less implant, memories in their subjects (Freud, 1896; Levis, 1990).

However, Loftus (1993) notes that memories in storage may become an amalgam of "borrowed ideas, characters, myths, accounts from exogenous sources with idiosyncratic internal beliefs," perhaps serving as screens for "more prosaic but, ironically, less tolerable, painful experiences of childhood" (pp. 524–525). Memories also can be altered by shifts in modalities in storage, as supplemental information presented in an auditory mode can transfer into or alter a visual image, even if no visual encoding has occurred (Loftus, 1979; Loftus & Christianson, 1989). Memories also may be changed in storage through "motivated overwriting" wherein retroactive interference (e.g., interference by emotions, events, or interpretations after the traumatic event) allows burial of a specific association by emotionally motivated attempts to "cover it" with different, affectively incompatible associations (Bower, 1990, p. 220; Lehman &

Bovasso, 1993). These and other misinformation effects will be considered in some detail later in the section on suggestibility.

RETRIEVAL

Retrieval may also provide an explanation for forgetting or inaccessibility of early memories. A number of factors can affect retrieval. One consideration already discussed concerns the socialization processes by which a child learns how to remember through adult provision of retrieval cues enabling the learning of retrieval strategies (Hudson, 1990; Neisser, 1990; Nelson, 1988; Ratner et al., 1990; Schachtel, 1959). Retrieval strategies alone, however, may be necessary but not sufficient for recall of certain early events. Due, perhaps, to limits in schematic organization, lingual ability, and effective search–recall strategies, episodic memories encoded during childhood may be dependent on highly specific context and cues for adequate retrieval (Erdelyi, 1990; Myers et al., 1994; Rovee-Collier & Shyi, 1992; Spiegel et al.,1993). It may be that memories survive storage, with more or less modification or distortion, but the encoding context (both internally and externally) is discrepant from the retrieval context, making recall difficult or impossible. Such discrepancies may be related to differences in cue salience between early childhood and adulthood (i.e., elements of the experience salient to and encoded by a young child may be quite different from aspects of an experience considered salient and memorable by an adult). In addition, the meaning of an experience likely changes from early childhood to adulthood, creating consider-able difficulty in reestablishing a context with adequate retrieval cues to aid in recall (Bauer, 1995; Howe & Courage, 1993; Myers et al., 1994; Pillemer & White, 1989).

In suggesting that most memory impairment is related to retrieval, Bower (1990) has noted that memories do not "go anywhere; memories are simply dispositions that can be actualized in certain circumstances (or retrieval environments) and not in others. They are like 'responses' waiting for the right 'stimulus' to release them" (p. 222). The specificity of the stimulus or cue needed for memory retrieval increases with age and retention interval as does the use of contextual information (Howe & Courage, 1993). As trauma can incorporate distinctive cues, including highly intense emotions not often represented in normal human experience, reestablishment of a fully appropriate retrieval context may be unlikely.

These ideas correspond to a theory of state-dependent memory described as early as 1892 by Janet who noted that remembering depends on the "state of the subject at the moment when he acquires the remembrance" as well as the "state of the subject when he tries to reproduce the remembrance" (p. 106). It may be that an alteration in state alters the context and thus the functional retrieval cues (Christianson & Nilsson, 1989; Liwag & Stein, 1995; Swanson & Kinsbourne, 1979). Traumatic dissociative amnesia might even be considered an extreme form of state-dependent memory involving body sensations, physiological states, emotions, and other key retrieval cues (Janet, 1892; Putnam, 1991; Spiegel, 1990). Emotional states, in particular, are thought to be powerful retrieval links to episodic memory, especially if the specific emotion is perceived as causally related to the event being recalled (Liwag & Stein, 1995). However, if aversive affective states are avoided, as may be the case with trauma, retrieval may be difficult, even in the presence of other cues (Bower, 1990; Liwag & Stein, 1995; Spiegel et al., 1993). An individual must be willing and able to tolerate the reexperiencing of traumatic emotion if successful episodic retrieval is to occur. Semantic or procedural memories of a traumatic event may be retained because they are dissociated from conscious comprehension and emotional activation. If the episodic memory of the trace-producing event is retrieved, it may stimulate the emotional memory as well (Greenwald, 1992). If retrieval does, in fact, activate an emotional state linked to the trauma, defense maneuvers to reduce affective distress may be triggered, shifting the state and aborting successful retrieval (Greenberg & van der Kolk, 1987). Even if defensive maneuvers do not alleviate the emotional arousal, some cognitive resources will be directed toward this arousal state, still limiting conscious attention and hindering the resources available to the retrieval process (Christianson & Nilsson, 1984).

A shift in consideration toward the parallel distributed processing or network model would suggest that retrieval efforts will be determined by associative links between various features of a memory as well as by the integration of the network over which the memory features are distributed. The memory network includes a constellation of features including "feelings, attributes, properties, and causal sequences of scenes, each of which can serve as an 'index cue' for recalling more or less of the constellation" (Bower, 1990, p. 221). The availability of appropriate index cues and the strengths of the linkages between them will determine retrieval success. Further, to access a complete network as a unit, according to this theory, a critical number of features must match input information, internal associations, or both (McNally, 1993). However, with trauma, the associative network can be expansive, as respondent conditioning can pair a large array of cues to the original traumatic stimulus properties. Over time, this fear network can expand as new cues are paired with retraumatizing intrusive recall. Retrieval then may result in indiscriminate activation of the network, as well as excess information being accessed, making retrieval efforts vulnerable to interference by a large number of other associative pathways that may be activated (Christianson & Nilsson, 1984). This process might, in part, explain the enhanced startle response, flashbacks, and other intrusive symptomatology often seen in trauma survivors.

SUGGESTIBILITY

Particularly in a discussion of traumatic memory, the question of suggestibility often arises. To what degree are memories veridical, more or less naturally distorted or lost, or distorted through suggestion of various sorts? Although many of the mechanisms considered earlier can be applied to this question, a discussion specific to the literature on suggestibility seems warranted. First, however, it may be important to determine a working definition of suggestibility. Ceci and Bruck (1993) define suggestibility as concerning the degree to which "encoding, storage, retrieval, and reporting of events can be influenced by a range of social and psychological factors" (p. 404). Thus this definition allows that suggestibility may have both cognitive factors and factors related to social demands. Various hypotheses have been offered to account for such effects. These include the following: (1) an original trace is overwritten by erroneous information; (2) the original trace remains intact but is rendered unretrievable due to access competition; (3) original details are not attended to and thus not encoded, allowing erroneous information to fill gaps in the trace; (4) difficulty with source monitoring enhances the likelihood of incorporating erroneous information; and (5) social pressures lead to the reporting, rehearsal, and possibly eventual incorporation of erroneous information (Ceci & Bruck, 1993).

The first hypothesis implies trace erasure or alteration in which the original trace is distorted beyond recognition and thus cannot be retrieved (Zaragoza, Dahlgren, & Muench, 1992). Related to trace strength, this effect may occur as misinformation degrades the memory by either distorting the trace or interfering with retrieval, or both. Toglia and colleagues (1992) have noted that "the degree of degradation is a monotonic function of the current strength of memory for the original event" (p. 232). Further, the retroactive interference literature offers support for this idea of greater suggestibility with weak traces (Zaragoza et al., 1992). Specifically, it may be that with weaker traces, misinformation is more readily accepted because no competing trace challenges the suggestion (Ceci & Bruck, 1993).

However, there is some debate as to whether or not traces are actually erased. Zaragoza and colleagues (1992) and others have found little unequivocal evidence of actual erasure or degradation of original traces. Rather, they have demonstrated misinformation effects without such impairment effects across a wide range of experiments. Thus it has been suggested that all traces survive, though at different strengths, allowing a coexistence of the original traces with the misinformation traces. As such, new (e.g., postevent) information does not necessarily modify previously stored events but is stored in a separate, stronger trace or a trace of equal strength, creating response competition during retrieval. However, postevent misinformation traces may be stronger due to recency effects or increased saliency if attention has been drawn to the misinformation by an authority figure, further weakening a relatively weak original trace (Toglia et al., 1992). This may be a particular issue in children, who tend toward formation of more impoverished representations, leaving them more susceptible to misinformation effects in the decreased likelihood that they will detect discrepancies. Additionally, children, in general, tend to forget more than adults. Thus memory weakens more rapidly and is thereby more susceptible to misinformation (Loftus, Hoffman, & Wagenaar, 1992).

Related to children's tendency to create impoverished traces, the possibility exists that certain aspects of an experience simply are not encoded, leaving an open door for misinformation to fill gaps in the trace. Therefore, if a detail is left unencoded, misinformation aimed at that aspect of the experience may simply be accepted as "true" given that no response competition exists to create any internal discrepancy (Zaragoza et al., 1992).

This would most likely be true for peripheral detail rather than essence, however.

Another possibility involves difficulties with source monitoring, which involves "discriminating memories that originated from perception from those that arose from thought, imagination, fantasy, dreams and other self-generated processes" (Johnson, 1991, p. 6). Source monitoring problems can occur when one confuses the origin of information, misattributing something that was reflectively generated to perception or vice versa. Problems with source monitoring may also be exacerbated when the decision criteria for determining the reality or veracity of a given memory are relaxed (e.g., when a suggestion is made to accept as true any image, thought, or dream that occurs in a client suspecting abuse) (Ceci & Loftus, 1994).

Perhaps related to original trace strength and other individual factors, the difficulties with source monitoring do not necessarily imply memory impairment. It is widely believed that such difficulties reflect, particularly in children, fragile boundaries between fantasy and reality that may be further blurred with intense emotion. Specifically, children may have less developed abilities for differentiating between actual and imagined events in some cases, particularly when one of the information sources is self-generated or when the sources of information are perceptually and semantically similar (Ceci & Bruck, 1993; Ceci, Huffman, Smith, & Loftus, 1994; Lindsay & Read, 1994). However, some empirical research challenges the extent of source monitoring difficulty in children, suggesting instead that children possess relatively sophisticated memory abilities that frequently preclude such distortions (Fivush, 1994b; Toglia et al., 1992). In either children or adults, though, difficulties with source monitoring may have less to do with the sophistication of memory than with the creation of additional competing traces. Specifically, it may be that simple repetition of misinformation, questions including misinformation, or imagined events can over time create a trace that is difficult to distinguish from an actual historical memory (Lindsay & Read, 1994).

Finally, social demand characteristics may enhance the likelihood of misinformation or suggestibility effects. At any age, conformity to perceived social pressure can increase the tendency to report misinformation, even though the original memory remains intact (Zaragoza et al., 1992). In addition, a "prestige effect" can occur, involving the attribution of credibility to an authority figure giving misinformation (Lindsay & Read, 1994; Toglia et al,. 1992, p. 223). Children are thought in some cases to be particularly susceptible to such social pressure, as some studies have found misinformation effects to be stronger with adult confederates supplying erroneous information than with peer confederates supplying the same misinformation to children (Toglia et al., 1992). It appears that, in many cases, children perceive adults as cooperative, truthful, and unlikely to be deceptive as well as credible and competent sources of information (Ceci & Bruck, 1993). This tendency to trust adult perceptions over their own may combine with the proclivity of young children to comply with and please authority figures in enhancing suggestibility effects. Various studies have supported this hypothesis (Ceci & Bruck, 1993; Lindsay & Read, 1994). Even in adults, perceived authority may enhance suggestibility.

Particularly in traumatic situations, these social demands can be particularly potent. Since humans, especially at young ages, depend on the perceptions and beliefs of others to validate their own reality testing, denial or invalidation by others creates a withdrawal of social support that can disrupt beliefs, perceptions, and self-trust. Particularly with traumatic events that themselves can seem unreal and nonveridical in their departure from normal human experience, a lack of social validation may significantly affect memory, contributing not only to suggestibility but also to forgetting (Waites, 1993). Also related, Loftus and Kaufman (1992) consider the secondary gains afforded in a context of social pressure to produce or alter memories, particularly if suggestion is provided by an authority figure. For example, if a therapist confidently suggests the existence of trauma as explanatory for various symptoms in a client, the client may be susceptible to suggestion given perceived authority of the therapist. Or in contrast, if an authority figure invalidates or attempts to alter a child's own perceptions of a traumatic event, the status of the memory for that event may be affected. Thus in a context of malicious (vs. accidental) trauma, erroneous interpretations or "forgetting" may be reinforced by a perpetrator who uses threats or other coercive means to ensure the victim's silence (Enns et al., 1995).

Although most of the above hypotheses consider age differences, with young children believed to be more suggestible than adults, the existence of clear, linear age effects in suggestibility has not been unequivocally demonstrated. Rather, age may interact with other factors known to increase suggestibility in complex ways that influence degree of suggestibility. These factors include repetition and number of suggestions, retention interval, linguistic complexity of misleading information, plausibility of misinformation, emotional salience of the original event, degree of schematic development in the child, relation of the original event to the degree of elaboration of the relevant schema, degree of reliance on schematized knowledge, and others (Ceci & Bruck, 1993; Ceci et al., 1994; Garry, Loftus, & Brown, 1994; Lindsay & Read, 1994).

Regardless of age, some of these factors are especially potent, including the degree of repetition, plausibility of misinformation, and retention interval, all factors of considerable salience in psychotherapy with an adult suspecting early trauma. However, even in children, studies have found that central information is difficult to alter, particularly in high-stress situations, and degree of prior knowledge of an event may mitigate the degree of suggestibility (Ceci & Bruck, 1993; Goodman et al., 1991; Goodman et al., 1994; Pezdek & Roe, 1994). Further, while details, particularly peripheral details, may be susceptible to misinformation effects, the possibility of creating, through suggestion, entire memories never experienced is questionable, and little systematic research supports such a phenomenon (Berliner & Williams, 1994; Enns et al., 1995; Goodman et al., 1991; Harvey & Herman, 1994; Pezdek, 1994; Pezdek & Roe, 1994), even though such effects have been reported in anecdotal and qualitative reports (e.g., Ceci et al., 1994; Garry et al., 1994; Lindsay & Read, 1994). Finally, one additional factor in considering misinformation effects suggests that the potential for suggestibility is greater when the topic of suggestion is of little personal concern, a situation inconsistent with suggestibility for personal trauma (Pezdek, 1994).

In any configuration, however, it is most often extremely difficult to distinguish misinformation from actual (veridical) memory, as distorted memories may be "highly vivid, internally coherent, and contain many low-frequency perceptual details" (Ceci & Loftus, 1994, p. 355). Thus no particular attributes of a given memory can be used to determine its veracity, and the ability of even professionals to make such distinctions is demonstrably poor (Lindsay & Read, 1994; Neisser, 1994; Terr, 1994).

Schema Theory and Integrative Models

The previous discussion, while heuristically useful, suggests artificial breaks in what is currently thought to be a continuous functioning of the memory system. A careful reading will, in fact, reveal the difficulty in separating out mutually exclusive functions of encoding, storage, and retrieval. However, broader models integrate these processes in understanding memory functioning, suggesting an interplay between multiple memory processes in determining the nature of traumatic memory. To demonstrate this interplay in very simplistic terms: a traumatic event must first be registered and interpreted, with selective attention likely to inhibit affect-laden contents or restrict elaborative processing. Then during encoding at various levels, the information must be transmitted to the brain, interpreted first perceptually, then associated and organized for storage if, in fact, a relevant schema can be matched to the traumatic event. For recall, the effectiveness of a given retrieval cue is dependent upon what has been perceived, encoded, and stored, with the initial restrictions of attention possibly resulting in a paucity of associative connections available for retrieval (Bonanno, 1990a; Christianson & Nilsson, 1984; Spiegel et al., 1993; Swanson & Kinsbourne, 1979). Parallel distributed processing (PDP) network and schema theories may offer an integrated means of considering such complexity in the memorial system in trauma, as the data-driven (or bottom-up) nature of the PDP networks work in concert with the concept-driven (or top-down) schemas (Spiegel et al., 1993).

The complex networks specified by PDP theory may be arranged hierarchically with subnetworks nested within supraordinate networks of larger meaning systems. Memories may be understood as clusters of attributes organized such that processing a particular concept can activate the most closely related concepts, and through spreading activation, eventually make the entire constellation of related concepts available for decision processes (Sheffield & Hudson, 1994). The supraordinate networks, much like psychological schemas, process information in parallel, sequentially accessing a central processor (i.e., active consciousness). Memories consist of a pattern of interrelationships activated by perceptual input that binds the subunits at certain levels of "mutual excitation and inhibition" (Bauer, 1995; Greenwald, 1992; Spiegel, 1990, p. 122; see also Stinson & Palmer, 1991). Dynamic and perseverative cycles of activation occur, consolidating and elaborating memories in storage, with new information able, in most cases, to cause accommodation of the relative weights or bonds within the net.

The strength of the bonds and the rules for organization and interaction between subunits in the network will determine the degree of integration or the degree of dissociation between these subunits in storage, affecting later efforts at retrieval. Ideally, a unitary consciousness will span and merge the various networks, much like a computer's central processing unit (Spiegel, 1990; Neisser, 1990). This level of integration, in turn, determines the activation pathways stimulated with input, with a variable number of features of a memory retrieved with specified cues. This dynamic activation "stabilizes into a pattern that reflects input information and constraints embodied in the network of connections" (Stinson & Palmer, 1991, p. 353).

In other words, the schematic networks constrain the nature of perceiving and organizing information, while simultaneously the input activates specific pathways determined by— and perhaps defining—the schemas. Thus from this integrated model, schemas are "implicit structures distributed over the mass of interconnections" (Stinson & Palmer, 1991, p. 353). The networks, with their interconnecting bonds, carry the ability when activated to generate states that correspond to "instantiated schemas," which exist as specific activation patterns of the net (Stinson & Palmer, 1991, p. 353). Thus both initial encoding as well as memory retrieval involve a cue that reinstates a net activation pattern, or a schema.

The effects of trauma on such a system, then, are far-reaching. First, trauma may disrupt the integration necessary to the unified functioning of the complex networks. Particularly, repeated traumatic events may result in a disruption in network (i.e., schema) formation, resulting in discrete, isolated pathways unintegrated and unconnected by a unified consciousness. The intensity of emotional arousal may contribute to strong, exclusive bonds within a trauma network that further contribute to its isolation. There also may be an all-or-none activation pattern, corresponding loosely to the posttraumatic stress intrusion and denial phases outlined by Horowitz (1988). This can leave the schematic network fixed and maladaptive and can make memory retrieval either vivid and intrusive, depending on the size of the associative network of cues, or difficult in the case of a specified, narrow, unelaborated pathway. Further the disruption of network (schema) formation may significantly alter the encoding and storage of later information (including repetition of traumatic events) (McCann & Pearlman, 1990).

Horowitz (1988) conceptualizes the functioning of memory for trauma from an integrated frame combining psychodynamic and cognitive theories in a model compatible with cognitive PDP theory just discussed. This model integrates the processing of external sensory input with internal schemas and memory networks in considering a synthesized composite schematic representation. In general, traumatic experiences lie outside the existing memory networks, or schemas, and thus cannot be assimilated into the networks even if they achieve adequate encoding. Thus these representations remain in an active memory store (outside the long-term networks or schemas) that is perseverative in its repeated representation of traumatic event features in various modalities. The repeated representation alternates with inaccessibility caused by cognitive and emotional control processes that titrate the degree of activation and arousal, allowing processing to occur in a modulated, adaptive manner. Through this process, the features of the traumatic memory are continually recoded and reinterpreted in an iterative process that eventually either forges pathways for assimilation or pathways isolated outside established networks and prone to earlier decay (Horowitz, 1988).

A child with unformed or newly formed networks, or schemas, may stabilize psychological experience by compartmentalizing the activation pathways (or subschemas) to organize the information in manageable subunits, resulting in a developmental dissociation in processes and networks. The lack of integration allows only one subschema or subunit access to consciousness at a time. Horowitz (1988) notes that in this way "self-coherence is protected at the expense of developing realistic working models" (p. 107).

It should be noted, in the spirit of integrative thinking, that these theories of cognitive science are fully compatible with current thinking in clinical dissociation theory. Specifically, one of the theories of dissociation previously discussed includes the notion

> that the mental apparatus consists of a set of cognitive structures similar to Janet's automatisms and Bartlett's (1932) schemata, which monitor, organize, and control both thought and action in various domains. Each of these structures can seek or avoid inputs, facilitate or inhibit outputs. The structures are arranged hierarchically . . . are normally in communication . . . and are linked to a superordinate structure that provides for executive monitoring and control. As the ultimate endpoint for all inputs, and the ultimate starting point for all outputs, the executive control structure provides the psychological basis for the phenomenal experiences of awareness and intentionality. However, certain conditions can alter the integration and organization of these structures, breaking the links between one or more subsystems or between a subsystem and the executive. Such a situation results in a condition of divided consciousness, in which percepts, thoughts, feelings, and actions are processed without being represented in phenomenal awareness. (Kihlstrom, 1990, p. 455)

This summary of dissociative processes is strikingly similar to the concepts proffered in PDP theory as well as those suggested in schema theory.

Summary: Cognitive Processes in Traumatic Memory

As is apparent, the actual cognitive processes of memory functioning are complex, and trauma serves only to increase this complexity. Although any number of processes can be used to understand traumatic memory, it is most likely that this phenomenon is multiply determined, with various cognitive factors interacting with individual differences in development, personality, and environmental circumstances. In addition, it may be that traumatic memory is more similar than dissimilar to "normal" memory processing.

However, it may be helpful to attempt to distill the complexity into a conclusive strand of thought. In sum, it seems that traumatic experience in early childhood can be, and most often is, accurately "remembered" in one or more memory modalities, as memory in childhood appears to be relatively well developed. For example, if early memories are encoded nonverbally, they may be retrieved and accurately expressed nonverbally, but outside verbal comprehension (Howe & Courage, 1993). It is essential to recognize, then, that memory can exist in other than verbal forms, although verbal modalities may be essential to achieving full conscious awareness and recall. However, various developmental processes may prevent the retention of very early memories for adult recall. Specifically, a combination of factors ranging from detail and strength of memory traces, to facility with language relative to verbal encoding and social communication, to the development of a self-structure capable of sustaining episodic, autobiographical memory may preclude full, verbal encoding and recall of early events.

However, where memories are encoded and potentially available, other specific cognitive mechanisms may interfere. Encoding, storage, and retrieval processes all may serve as underlying mechanisms by which early traumatic memories are rendered inaccessible for later recall due to various factors such as selective or narrowed attention, degree of emotional arousal, and accurate matching of encoding and retrieval contexts and cues. Further, these specific mechanisms may interact with large schematic structures or networks in traumatic memory. For example, threat to schematic integrity may interfere with encoding, storage, and retrieval processes. Further, although memory for one-time traumatic events may remain more or less intact, memory for repeated traumas may suffer greater distortion due to schematic and network processing. Specifically, repeated traumas may be fused into generalized schematic representations that are separated from larger associative networks. Moreover, even for single traumas, if schemas, or associative networks, do not provide a match for incoming traumatic information, the encoding of the trauma may be forged into an isolated pathway unable to be connected, by either assimilation or accommodation, to larger nets. Thus full retrieval may be difficult, although activation of the traumatic pathway may occur with or without larger associative meaning contexts.

These processes may provide the cognitive underpinnings of dissociative processes. Such processes may contribute to differential encoding of experiences leading to unintegrated network pathways. However, application of cognitive mechanisms to the phenomenon of repression may be less fruitful. Repression per se may be a less parsimonious explanation for what, in essence, may be disruption in accessibility to traumatic memories caused by any of various cognitive mechanisms. Despite the fact that repression has been subject to much debate and refutation (Holmes, 1990), its refutation does not nullify the existence of motivated forgetting, as has been suggested. It is clear that forgetting, motivated and otherwise, does occur, and it may occur as a result of highly specific and complex cognitive processes interacting with emotional states. Or, more specifically, what is termed repression may simply be an absence of accessibility of verbal or symbolic memory, even in the presence of memories in other modalities—a sort of remembering without awareness. This explanation would not be inconsistent with Freud (1915a) or Janet (1892) in their understanding of the necessary verbal component for consciousness. Therefore the debate and controversy over motivated forgetting in terms of repression may be one reflecting semantic distinctions more than anything else. As such, it may be more precise to consider the distortion or forgetting of traumatic material in terms of the probable mechanisms involved rather than in the recondite phenomenon of repression.

Neurophysiological Substrates of Traumatic Memory

Although memory has been the subject of much theory and research in neurophysiological laboratories for more than a century, only recently have such efforts been devoted to the neurophysiological substrates of traumatic memory. Both theory and research in this area are complex and, in some areas, speculative. However, research with human and nonhuman primates is increasingly providing an empirical base in support of the developing theory. Although the complexity of this body of research precludes a detailed and exhaustive examination here, a brief overview of the literature will provide an interesting integration with psychological and cognitive theories discussed.

Neurological Development and Memory

In considering the fate of childhood experiences in long-term memory, it may be that neurological maturation plays a role in rendering early episodic experiences less accessible than later experiences. A number of hypotheses are reviewed briefly below. (The supporting studies are not detailed but are noted in the references.)

MYELINIZATION AND THE LIMBIC SYSTEM

Myelinization of areas of the brain associated with learning and memory has been implicated in the decreased accessibility of childhood memories. Specifically, myelinization of the hippocampus, thought to be an essential neurological structure in memory, and the hippocampal localization system, which fixes episodic memories in a proper context in time and space, is incomplete in the first few years of life, perhaps leaving early memories without adequate context cues for retrieval. However, the taxon system, which processes memories in terms of their quality (i.e., feel or sound) develops much earlier. Thus details of early experiences may be inaccessible, but the quality of early experiences accessible, in long-term memory (van der Kolk, Boyd, Krystal, & Greenberg, 1984). Further, severe or prolonged stress can disrupt the hippocampal localization system, while potentiating the taxon system, leaving emotionally tinged memories that are context-free (Howe & Courage, 1993; van der Kolk et al., 1984; van der Kolk & van der Hart, 1991). In addition, activity in the hippocampus, rich in corticosteroid receptors selectively activated during stress, may be suppressed. Thus an attendant increase in corticosteroid levels might create amnesia for traumatic experiences. Memories, then, may be encoded only in sensorimotor forms and, therefore, difficult to translate into verbal forms (i.e., conceptual language) necessary for conscious verbal retrieval (van der Kolk et al., 1984).

Some studies suggest that the hippocampus is involved specifically with recent long-term events, while remote long-term storage may depend on elaboration of hippocampal connections to various functional systems in the brain, perhaps due to certain biochemical reactions or to rehearsal leading to an increase in interconnections (Khan, 1986). The development of connections between the hippocampus and the neocortex in particular may be associated with the development of remote long-term memory. In addition, the locus coeruleus (LC), which is associated with activation of fear responses and memory formation, projects into the cerebral cortex, the hippocampus, the amygdala, the hypothalamus, and the thalamus and may be strongly involved in remote long-term memory consolidation (Hartman & Burgess, 1993; Khan, 1986). Experiences in early life, particularly traumatic experiences, may be rendered uninterpretable and unelaborated due to immaturity of hippocampal connections to the neocortex and the amygdaloid complex.

Further the hippocampus is part of the larger corticolimbic system that is thought to be related to episodic memory storage. (A separate system—the corticostriatal system—is associated with semantic memory and is thought to mature earlier than the corticolimbic system.) Bauer (1995) cites various studies finding that damage to the limbic system interferes with declarative memory formation as well as with short-term memory retrieval. Further, studies with animals have shown that maturation (including myelinization and synaptogenesis) of this system is related to improvements in memory task performance. As the cortex and limbic areas can function somewhat independently in processing verbal comprehension and affective response respectively, immature synaptic efficiency may be related to the dissociation of strong emotional memories from verbal episodic memories (Weinberger, 1990). Howe and Courage (1993) conclude that "the pervasive human inability to recall experiences during infancy may well be a natural consequence of the immaturity of the corticolimbic system early in ontogeny" (p. 310).

PREFRONTAL CORTEX

The immaturity of the prefrontal cortex is also thought to be related to memory loss for early events. Specifically, in the first 2 years of human life (specifically 8 to 24 months), a rapid synaptogenesis occurs in the prefrontal cortex, coinciding with enhancement of a variety of cognitive tasks including memory. The increased synaptic density during this time may facilitate access, use, and behavioral application of stored information represented in memory, and this process may be refined over development through subsequent decreases in synaptic density (a sort of "pruning"), continued myelinization, development of neurotransmitters, or improved synaptic efficiency (Howe & Courage, 1993, p. 311). Thus events occurring prior to 24 months of age may lack adequate storage and elaboration due to immaturity of the prefrontal cortex.

LONG-TERM POTENTIATION

Finally, mastery of developmental tasks can catalyze biochemical reactions that lead to long-term potentiation (LTP), which involves lasting structural changes in synaptic connections, strengthening these connections, and enhancing the efficiency and speed of processing in the potentiated neuronal pathways (Carlson, 1991; Charney, Deutch, Krystal, Southwick, & Davis, 1993). Potentiation of neuronal pathways, particularly noradrenergic pathways projecting to the amygdala, may be related to the enhanced encoding of vivid trauma memories, which may remain susceptible to modulating influences (e.g., storage and retrieval enhancement) long after the initial acquisition (Charney et al., 1993; McGaugh, Introini-Collison, Naghara, & Cahill, 1989).

LTP, which is known to be related to learning, occurs readily in the hippocampal formation and may serve as a specific biological substrate to memory. Studies have demonstrated the occurrence of LTP with mastery of certain cognitive tasks and have shown that the LTP capability of the hippocampal region increases with age in animals (Howe & Courage, 1993). Howe and Courage (1993) conclude in a review of developmental and neurological literature that, while no evidence supports theories of developmental discontinuity, there are "neurological constraints that probably set limits on how well infants perceive, learn, and remember, particularly in the first year of life" (p. 312). These constraints, particularly in interaction with traumatic experience, may contribute to a disruption in memory functioning in early trauma.

Trauma and the Neurobiology of Memory

Beyond these developmental constraints affecting memory for early events, trauma seems to initiate specific neurophysiological responses that may alter memory functioning. These involve biochemical reactions and their subsequent effects on potentiation and elaboration of neural pathways.

CATECHOLAMINE SYSTEM, AROUSAL, AND LTP

The LC, known to be structurally significant in memory functioning, activates the central nervous system during threat. When the LC is activated, catecholamines (norepinephrine, dopamine, and serotonin) are released. The release of these neurotransmitters leads to autonomic arousal (with its enhanced vigilance and attentiveness to stimuli) as well as hyperpotentiation of noradrenergic neuronal pathways (by enhancing neuronal response) from the LC to the hippocampus, amygdala, thalamus, and frontal lobes where interpretation of danger further enhances fight/flight/freeze behavioral responses. Some research has shown, in fact, that lesions to the specified pathways can interrupt posttraumatic stress symptoms such as enhanced startle (Charney et al., 1993). In regard to early memory, the neocortical components and the reciprocal connections between the hippocampus and the neocortex are thought to develop later than the hippocampus thus compromising the ability for organized long-term retention of episodic memories (see studies cited in Bauer, 1995).

Specific responses associated with trauma-induced states of high arousal (such as focused attention and hypervigilance) at optimal levels may enhance memory consolidation of the traumatic event (although such consolidation may result in a memorial constellation that is encapsulated and isolated from other memory contents) (Bremner, Davis, Southwick, Krystal, & Charney, 1993). Charney and colleagues (1993) suggest that "emotional memories established via thalmoamygdala pathways may be relatively indelible" (p. 295). Pitman (1989) refers to this process as "superconditioning," resulting from the neurochemically induced overconsolidation of a memory trace (p. 222). However, an inverted–U-shaped dose–response curve suggests that at exceedingly high levels of stress-related neurochemical activity, memory consolidation may be inhibited, leading to amnesias (Pitman, 1989). This is consistent with certain cognitive research findings that have demonstrated a similar relationship between arousal level and memory.

The intense arousal of inescapable trauma quickly causes neurotransmitter use to exceed synthesis, depleting the catecholamines released and resulting in a hypersensitivity (perhaps due to receptor upregulation) to these neurotransmitters. Studies with animals have shown that once neuronal pathways have been activated by severe stress, these pathways are potentiated such that subsequent stress of lesser intensity or perceived threat will preferentially activate the same pathways, potentially, and at times indiscriminately, activating memories laid down previously in trauma. The amygdala with its extensive connections to cortical sensory systems may also contribute to this hypersensitivity. Specifically, traumatic memories may eventually be stored in the cortex rather than the amygdala and may be susceptible to reactivation by sensory stimuli with any functional interchange between the sensory cortices (where memories of each sense may be stored) and the amygdala (Charney et al., 1993; McGaugh et al., 1989; see Bauer, 1995, for review of other studies).

After repeated traumas, even associated states or contextual cues can stimulate excessive noradrenergic release onto the hypersensitive system, further potentiating these pathways (particularly those from the LC or medial geniculate body to the hippocampus or amygdala) and leading to intense, often eidetic but fragmented reexperience. Related to state-dependent memory as well as dissociative processes, this neurological process may contribute to the initiation of the intrusive reliving of traumatic events in flashbacks or nightmares (Burgess & Hartman, 1992; Charney et al., 1993; Chemtob, Roitblat, Hamada, Carlson, & Twentyman, 1988; Hartman & Burgess, 1993; Putnam, 1991; Schetky, 1990; van der Kolk & Greenberg, 1987; van der Kolk & van der Hart, 1991; Waites, 1993; Wilson, 1989).

A further memory effect occurs with the interaction of noradrenergic levels and memory for repeated traumas. Specifically, a depletion in noradrenergic levels may decrease memory functioning, while an increase in noradrenergic substances at certain optimal levels may enhance memory. Effects on memory then may vary with the phases of the biochemical trauma response, perhaps explaining the observed phenomenon of single-trauma memory enhancement and repeated-trauma memory impairment. Specifically, single trauma may stimulate noradrenergic release, whereas repeated trauma also stimulates opioid release, which, in turn, suppresses the release of norepinephrine (Chemtob et al., 1988; McGaugh et al., 1989; Putnam, 1991; Schetky, 1990; van der Kolk et al., 1984; van der Kolk & Greenberg, 1987; van der Kolk & van der Hart, 1991; Waites, 1993; Wilson, 1989). However, this pattern is slightly more complex, in that the memory enhancement associated with higher levels of noradrenergic substances is limited as demonstrated by the dose–response curve that typically manifests as an inverted-U-shaped function. Beyond certain optimal levels, increases in noradrenergic levels actually may interfere with consolidation of memories, resulting in posttraumatic amnesia (Khan, 1986; Pitman, 1989).

ENDOGENOUS OPIOIDS

A second biochemical system significant in neurophysiological trauma response is the endogenous opioid system. This system responds specifically to duration or repetition of trauma, providing an analgesic or tranquilizing effect that is hypothesized to become physiologically addictive. The release of these substances is correlated with hypoarousal, constriction, numbing, escape deficits, and withdrawal (all of which also result from catecholamine depletion common in chronic trauma) (van der Kolk et al., 1984; van der Kolk & Greenberg, 1987; Waites, 1993). The numbing phase associated with endogenous opioids is related to memory impairment, perhaps caused in part by inhibition of the catecholamine system as well as by other effects of opioid numbing such as restricted attention, disruptions in cognitive processing and efficiency, and dissociative processes (Khan, 1986; McGaugh et al., 1989; Pitman, 1989; van der Kolk & Greenberg, 1987).

GLUCOCORTICOIDS

Studies with animals find that extreme stress results in significant increases in glucocorticoid levels in the brain. Sustained release of glucocorticoids in animals exposed to acute stress has been associated with damage to or loss of hippocampal neurons. Neuronal damage includes changes in cell architecture and increased vulnerability to other neurochemicals. Such changes in brain regions critical to memory functioning may be implicated in memory alterations (e.g., short-term memory functioning, amnesias, etc.) often seen accompanying trauma. Among other research findings supporting this hypothesis, studies with combat veterans with posttraumatic stress disorder showed a decrease in hippocampal volume compared with control subjects (Bremner et al., 1993; Khan, 1986).

NEURONAL NETWORKS

Related to the cognitive science PDP network model of memory, neuronal pathways, similar to associative pathways in PDP models, may be subsumed in larger matrices (similar to the concept of instantiated schema patterns) that function in a biochemically regulated parallel excitation–inhibition process. Certain pathways will be subject to excitation, while incompatible pathways are inhibited. Similar to the Horowitz (1988) model of traumatic memory, incoming information is maintained in a short-term activated state by perseverative reverberation of neural, electrical activity (the "labile phase"), until it achieves long-term structural or chemical storage (perhaps related to synaptic changes) in a "stable phase" (Khan, 1986, pp. 14–15). If trauma responses interfere with memory consolidation, this labile phase may continue to recycle memory traces, potentiating the traumatic pathways and disrupting the normal sequencing into stable memory (Khan, 1986).

In addition, a "spreading activation" of the traumatic, threat-arousal pathway may inadvertently activate corresponding pathways that then overload the cognitive system, potentiating behaviors and physiological responses that, in turn, affect subsequent neuronal potentiation (Chemtob et al., 1988, p. 266). This potentiation cycle then can affect trauma networks by creating higher "resting" levels of potentiation for threat-arousal and higher limits on the magnitude to which the traumatic pathway can be activated (Chemtob et al., 1988, p. 268). The pathways and activation patterns may be highly specific, resulting in an isolation or dissociation of the trauma network from other contents of memory, and retrievable only with distinct cues (Khan, 1986; Waites, 1993).

An additional result of this potentiation cycle may be increased rates of speed (or "gain") of the arousal feedback loop, resulting in enhanced sequences of perception of threat, threat arousal, and readiness to interpret information as threatening (Chemtob et al., 1988, p. 268). Specifically, incoming stimuli are transmitted from the limbic system along potentiated pathways in the neocortex where interpretation occurs. Since the arousal response originates in the limbic system (which can process perceptual and emotional information outside conscious [i.e., verbal] awareness), a dysregulation of this system resulting from the trauma cycles may compromise developing meaning networks or schemas in addition to consolidation of traumatic memories (Hartman & Burgess, 1993; Weinberger, 1990). A result of this disruption may be a dissociation between affect and verbal comprehension (Weinberger, 1990). Hartman and Burgess (1993) describe this as a "fundamental disruption in the integration of experiences. Behavior is separated from affect; affect from event; meaning is based on disrupted event processing" resulting in confusion of the meaning of information (p. 50).

KINDLING EFFECTS

In all of these cases, trauma may cause neurophysiological shifts to be enduring or permanent. For reasons not entirely understood, repetition of traumatic stress states (e.g., chronic traumatic events or a single traumatic event followed by intrusive reexperiences) can lead to lasting neurobiological changes due to a "kindling effect" (Hartman & Burgess, 1993; van der Kolk, 1987). In kindling studies, repeated intermittent electrical stimulations, too small to have singular effects, can, over time, produce major seizures and permanent alterations in neurological functioning. It is thought that such an effect in repeated, but unintegrated, representations of trauma may create such a kindling effect causing permanent alterations in neuronal pathways and neurochemical responses resulting in the endurance of biological sequelae of traumatic experiences.

Summary: Neurophysiology and Traumatic Memory

It is clear (more or less) in reviewing this complex body of literature that highly specific neuronal processes may be related to memory processes as understood psychologically or clinically. Specifically, both developmental (i.e., maturational) processes in the brain and specific neurochemical reactions triggered by traumatic experience have effects on the nature of memory for trauma. The developmental processes may contribute to the impairment of early memories in general, and traumatic memories in particular, due to immaturities in brain structures and neuronal pathways integral to memory consolidation. Further, trauma may trigger the release of certain neurochemicals that in some cases enhance memory consolidation and in others disrupt this process. Repeated trauma with its attendant biphasic neurochemical alterations may lead to greater impairments in memory, whereas memory for a single trauma may be neurochemically enhanced. Further, particularly intense or repeated trauma may result in long-term structural changes in the brain that continue to affect memory formation long after the offset of traumatic experience. Finally, neuronal networks may provide a substructure for cognitive memory network models (e.g., the PDP model), the understanding of which allows an integration of psychological, cognitive, and neurobiological factors in understanding memory for traumatic experience.

Therapeutic "Truth" of Memory for Trauma

Memory for trauma as related to dynamic mechanisms, schematic organization, specific cognitive mechanisms, and neurological processes is a complex psychological operation further complicated by the psychotherapeutic process of reconstruction of life narrative through interpersonal dialogue.

The interplay of these various factors, combined with environmental factors such as nature, duration, and threat of trauma, along with intrapsychic and developmental factors, create a matrix of possibilities sufficiently complex as to defy a simple and generalizable determination concerning "truth." However, the process of psychotherapy will be considered in relation to the various domains of memory in an attempt to clarify and understand these issues more fully.

Autobiographical Memory and Self

Memory for trauma may be assumed to belong specifically to autobiographical memory, which is a subsystem of episodic memory. Autobiographical memory is thought to comprise "the context, flow, and rhythm of daily life . . . the fabric of a self-knowledge system" (Barclay & DeCooke, 1988, p. 91). Bruhn (1990) also notes that autobiographical memory "provides an identity to the self, especially the self in relation to others and the world" (p. 41). Nelson (1993) describes autobiographical memory as "personal, long-lasting, and (usually) of significance to the self system. Phenomenally, it forms one's personal life history" (p. 8). Others also specify that autobiographical memory has a functional relationship to some aspect of self experience (Barclay, 1986; Barsalou, 1988; Brewer, 1986; Howe & Courage, 1993; Howe et al., 1994; Schachter, Kihlstrom, Kihlstrom, & Berren, 1989; Waites, 1993). As such, it may serve primarily to ensure continuity of subjective experience of self in the world. Specifically, the contents of autobiographical memory maintain a sense of congruence in self-knowledge, life themes, and sense of self (Barclay, 1986; Barclay & DeCooke, 1988). Thus "truth," as defined by objective history, is mediated by a sense of self and is "preserved at the expense of accuracy" to protect a consistent essence of self (Barclay, 1988, p. 298). In other words, since the content of autobiographical memory is intrinsically related to the experience of self and its integrity, memories are selectively true in the sense that they are understood or interpreted to affirm the self as understood and interpreted, while inconsistent details may be distorted or omitted in the interest of self-preservation. However, many believe there to be a fundamental integrity to most autobiographical memories (Enns et al., 1995), while others challenge this view (Neisser, 1994).

Just as the concept of self is debated as a true, emerging property of existence versus a socially constructed formation, the memories constituting the self may be subject to the same debate. Are autobiographical memories historically intact or constructed? And what are the implications for "truth" in either case? The weight of logical and empirical evidence would suggest a dialectic compromise between these two positions. Specifically, memories concerning self are inextricably linked to a sense of self that defines and is, in part, defined by these very memories as well as by the experiences that founded them.

Considering these issues, Kirschner (1993) suggested that "the interweaving of psychic and historical 'facts' forms the fabric of a subject who is not a unity but an open system, continually being redefined by new experiences and reinterpretations of the past, which in turn may highlight episodes previously forgotten or disregarded" (p. 228). Others (Brewer, 1986; Morris, 1993) add the solipsistic view that even basic perceptions are not "true" in the sense of objective truth but are interpreted at first registration by a perceiving self and its preconstructed categories of meaning. Bruner (1987) suggests that life as created by narrative is "a cognitive achievement" or an "interpretive feat" rather than a "through-the-clear-crystal recital of something univocally given" (p. 13). He notes that culturally influenced cognitive and linguistic processes structure perceptual experience and organize memory in creating autobiographical narratives that create a life and a self (Bruner, 1987). Such bias may relate to schematic screening of perception and recall as discussed earlier and may be similarly involved in individual differences in memory for trauma (Bonanno, 1990b; Bruhn, 1990). Thus in the moment of original experience as well as in recall, perceptions themselves are not infallibly veridical but are driven by a self.

Memories and their meanings, then, may be both reconstructed as well as constructed in that they are elaborated or transformed so the details fit into a life narrative in a manner consistent with the sense of self or the self-schema (Barclay, 1986, 1988; Bartlett, 1932; Bruhn, 1990; Bruner, 1994; Morris, 1993; Neisser, 1988; Tessler & Nelson, 1994). Thus the truth, as the self, is emergent as well as constructed. The relationship between autobiographical memory and the self is a "dynamic, interactive process in which self and memory organize, construct, and give meaning to each other in a way so intimate that we can truly say that we are what we remember and that our memories are ourselves" (Tessler & Nelson, 1994, p. 321). Barclay (1994) similarly describes autobiographical memory as an improvisational process through which a prototypical self is constructed and reconstructed through ongoing interactions with the world, other individuals, and one's own internal affective states. Thus a process of mutual influence occurs, in which self and experience interact in a manner that enables assimilation, accommodation, and continuity of experience. Weiser (1990) states this point cogently in her suggestion that "meaning doesn't really exist 'out there' apart from us, but rather it exists within the relationship between the object-stimulus and the person-perceiver" (p. 85).

Narrative Truth versus Historical Truth in Therapy

The nature of the question of truth, then, is altered, with a more relevant consideration focusing on the relative correspondence between event, perception, and memory in clarifying a life narrative, as well as the consistency of that narrative over time. Many suggest that therapy is a mutual process of calibrating this correspondence in a manner that provides an adaptive, functional, and consistent life narrative (Bartlett, 1932; Bonanno, 1990b; Gergen & Kaye, 1992; Morris, 1993; Neisser, 1994; Spence, 1982). In fact, Bruner (1987) considers the "principal function of mind" in general to be "world making" in the sense of narrative construction (p. 11). Thus, rather than recovering an objective past, clients, with their therapists, transcribe a personal history by subjectively structuring and reconfiguring a set of historical events (Bonanno, 1990b; Kirschner, 1993). Neisser (1994), in fact, suggests that memories are never simply observed by the client and later reported to the therapist, but rather are "constructs, shaped by the shared need to establish a psychoanalytically satisfactory narrative" (p. 6).

Even Freud, in spite of his occasional insistence of the historic accuracy of analytic reconstructions, recognized "the nature of our waking thought to establish order in material . . . , to set up relations in it and to make it conform to our expectations of an intelligible whole. . . . In fact, we go too far in this direction. . . . In our effort at making an intelligible pattern of the sensory impressions that are offered to us, we fall into the strangest errors" (1900, p. 499). Spence (1982) concurs, cautioning awareness of the distinction between historical-objective truth and narrative-constructed truth. Although the latter may retain the essence of the experience as it occurred, it is imbued with multiple biases. These biases emerge from the client in the telling, the therapist in the interpretation, and the constraints of a lingual representational system that requires linear coherence that can only roughly approximate phenomenal experience (Spence, 1982). Likewise, Weiser (1990) points out that we communicate primarily through language, but we must remember that language is only "*attempted representation*" for memories, feelings, and thoughts that are primarily iconic (p. 84).

Spence (1982) considers such issues in noting the preoccupation in the therapeutic setting with questions of truth and suggesting that therapists and clients acknowledge the impossibility of pure, objective truth given schematic biases in both perceiving and remembering. Rather, both therapist and client should allow for the utility of narrative truth based on the client–therapist constructive process as pragmatic, explanatory, and dynamic in the understanding and comprehension of life, experience, and self. However, these issues become more complex with the integration of traumatic experience into an autobiographical narrative.

Autobiographical Memory, Truth, and Trauma

Trauma inherently eludes comprehension, as most cultures provide few, if any, frames of thought or language to adequately structure traumatic experience. Thus, trauma may be selectively excluded from autobiographical memory due to its incongruence with self-schemas, normative expectations, and logical consistency with what "should" happen in one's life (Barclay & DeCooke, 1988). In addition, particularly with familial trauma, cultural and social scripts are significantly violated and tremendous loyalty conflicts engendered, rendering traumatic memory perhaps unacceptable for inclusion in a life narrative. Further, the avoidance of traumatic material due to emotional intensity may prevent its integration into a life narrative and disrupt autobiographical memory and thus self-integration, as discussed earlier (Terr, 1994; van der Hart et al., 1989; Waites, 1993). Indeed, the intensity of trauma may overwhelm psychological resources, temporarily fragmenting the functional boundaries of the ego and severing the traumatic events from an experiencing self (Laub & Auerhahn, 1993). The traumatic material may then become encapsulated with indelible memories existing in a trauma narrative separate from but parallel to the "normal" life narrative. As a result, a separate autobiographical memory store may contain only traumatic memories that are state-dependent and not integrated with the continuous life story defining the self. This can result in either a self-schema (or ego state) that remains unintegrated with subsequent experience, or the trauma can become an organizing and distorting focus in self-development. It is possible that the aftermath of trauma creates an alternation between an intact self with memory loss and a vivid traumatic memory with disturbed self-functioning (Waites, 1993).

Van der Kolk and van der Hart (1991), in interpreting Janet, distinguish normal narrative memory as social, variable across tellings, integrated and volitional, contextually based, and temporally ordered into a life history in contrast to the autistic, inflexible, unintegrated, decontextualized, and time-distorted nature of traumatic memory. Trauma may be "known" (through emotions, enactments, nightmares, fears, interpersonal patterns) but not consciously understood in the sense of narrative memory as identified. Thus trauma survivors often are "captive observers" who can only repeat the trauma but who cannot make sense of it, know it cognitively, or integrate it into a cohesive sense of self (Laub & Auerhahn, 1993, p. 288). To become part of the life narrative afforded by autobiographical memory, traumatic memory must be reworked and recategorized into coherent, socially communicable patterns that allow its placement in the life story (Laub & Auerhahn, 1993; van der Kolk & van der Hart, 1991). To become narrative, trauma must be transformed from a "knowing into telling" through verbal–lingual representation (Laub & Auerhahn, 1993, p. 288), and it must be subject to volitional recall and suppression.

It is this inclusion in the life narrative that is the subject of some debate. In order to be included in this narrative, must the traumatic material be completely accurate historically? Must it be verbally represented? If not encoded verbally, is it even possible that it may retain some level of truth in the transformation to language? Many suggest that narrative truth, whatever its form, is important in and of itself in the context of the client's meaning system, regardless of its degree of veracity. Others disagree, holding traumatic experience to a particularly stringent standard of truth and supporting corroboration of any traumatic material before its acceptance in the life narrative. Waites (1993) posits that particularly with trauma and its sequelae, the issue of truth is in some respects very salient. She says:

> Some therapists claim that psychological reality is all that matters anyway. But while this assumption highlights the

fact that experience is always interpreted and processed, it easily becomes a facile excuse for denying or glossing over the effects of real abuse. From a therapeutic standpoint, helping a victim to confront terrible and, at the time, uncontrollable realities as well as to distinguish between fantasy and reality is a necessary step in strengthening the capacity to exercise real adaptive control. (p. 36)

Ganaway (1989, 1991a, 1991b) echoes the need to consider the veracity of traumatic memory. He describes the child's use of fantasy to master untenable life experiences as well as "trance logic," which is used defensively and creates a logically inconsistent internal world characterized by primary process and preoperational cognitions (1989, p. 209). Although in childhood these maneuvers may be adaptive and developmentally appropriate, they are of little adaptive service in adult functioning. Further, trauma survivors often have intense self-doubt, questioning their own perceptions, sensory experiences, and interpretations (Kirschner, 1993). In order to achieve coherence and belief in self, coherence in memory is important. And for such coherence, perhaps both narrative memory and historic reality (to the extent that this can be captured) are necessary, as the therapist and client together reconstruct or reinterpret historical events within new frameworks of understanding, clarity, and meaning (Bonanno, 1990b; Kirschner, 1993). Although many believe that "strict veridicality is an illusion" (Bruhn, 1990, p. 66), some essence of truth or reality is possible, even in therapeutic reconstruction if a therapist is appropriately nondirective and nonsuggestive. Consequently, recognizing the constructive nature of the life narrative as defined or clarified through psychotherapy does not preclude the importance of considering the integrity of the process and its outcomes. Particularly where trauma is concerned, to do otherwise could be devastating. Beyond the need for basic corroboration, however, the real constraints of memory and narrative construction must be recognized and integrated in understanding traumatic memory in order to avoid a simplistic quest for "truth" as is often seen in legal settings.

The Integrative "Truth" of Trauma in Memory

The therapeutic dialogue—defined in part by the therapists' schemas, belief systems, biases, interpretations, and questions—presents a scaffolding for retrieval and comprehension of historical information much like that provided by adults surrounding the child learning how to remember. In the therapeutic space, as well as in any other life space, the various mechanisms of memory and perception cannot be divorced from such a social context in which meaning is created and validated (or invalidated as may be the case).

The very nature of the therapeutic dialogue might be understood to suggest that both experience and memory for experience are most likely shaped by intrinsic emergent qualities as well as by socially constructed meanings. Even at the point of initial sensory registration and perception, an actively constructing self is calling up schemas to direct attention and discern potential meanings. In this sense, we have no means to discern an objective truth, intrapsychically or interpersonally. Gergen and Kaye (1992) have noted that "narrative truth is to be distinguished from historical truth, and when closely examined, even the latter is found to be an imposter. What then is the function of narrative reconstruction? . . . to reorient the individual, to open new courses of action that are more fulfilling and more adequately suited to the individual's experiences, capacities, and proclivities" (p. 175). With this in mind, they refer to therapy as a dialogue through which occurs "the forging of meaning in the context of collaborative discourse" (p. 182).

Together, the therapist and client work to construct meaning from meaninglessness, to create continuity from chaos, and to instill empowerment and self-knowing from helplessness, all pertinent to the survivor of early trauma.

Thus the therapeutic dialogue in combination with individual differences and myriad cognitive, emotional, and neurological processes preclude definitive conclusions about whether each detail of a given memory for trauma is absolutely "true" as such. Rather, it is essential, though ultimately much more complicated, to leave this complexity intact in attempting to understand fully the individual survivor of traumatic experience. As such, the question of truth in psychotherapy may be directed most appropriately to considerations of integrity within the therapeutic relationship as well as within the individual therapist and individual client in terms of self-structure and life narrative. Mutuality in genuineness, honesty, and sincere collaborative striving for growth and healing create an openness to experience and understanding that, in its essence, can be relied upon to serve the best interests of the client and his or her search for truth. In such an environment, the question of truth may be answered most clearly by a subjective sense of fit and compatibility with the client's presentation and history. Such a fit is, perhaps, manifested in what Curtis (1991) describes as a "quiet knowing" that emerges over time in both therapist and client (p. 5). Within this frame, the life narrative is reconstructed in a way that enhances the emergence of the client's integrated, full self and provides a more sophisticated and complete knowing of the integrity of the client's truth and its function in ensuring integrity of the self.

Conclusions: Truth and Traumatic Memory

With this understanding, then, we can reconsider the various components of memory for trauma as articulated thus far. We know that accurate memory for early events is possible, and such memory may be retained over time if the memory is salient and/or rehearsed. However, trauma may affect normal memory processes emotionally, cognitively, and neurologically. Emotionally, defensive mechanisms, such as dissociation, can interfere with normal conscious processing of experience, leading to alterations in memory. While repression as a distinct phenomenon may have some role in memory for trauma, neither that role nor the nature of repression itself has yet been understood or identified clearly. Rather, repression may best be thought of less as a distinct phenomenon and more as a general representation of any of various cognitive mechanisms that interact with trauma to render memory inaccessible.

Specifically, trauma may present highly significant challenges to existing schemas of self and world, and the homeostatic regulation of schemas to ensure continuity as well as psychological and physical safety may present the "motivation" behind motivated forgetting. The need for schematic integrity may interact with dissociative processes to leave traumatic memory outside normal associative pathways and outside schematic organization. For early trauma, this may be, in part, related to immature cognitive processes, such as declarative memory, or it may be due to inadequate development of language, self-structure, and autobiographical memory systems. Further, the specific cognitive processes of encoding, storage, and retrieval may be disrupted as well, creating further insult to the capability to remember trauma with full accuracy and detail. As such, distributed processing networks that normally function in an integrated manner may be dysregulated such that alternate trauma-related networks remain isolated from a central interconnected network and executive processor. Dissociative processes may play a role in this disruption in the parallel distributed processing of consciousness and memory formation. Neurological substrates to this process may involve very specific neural and biochemical factors, including the potentiation and isolation of neuronal pathways and networks of activation.

In general then, despite the complexity, we can begin to see some convergence in elucidating the nature of traumatic memory from different windows of understanding. Specifically, dissociative processes either create pronounced divisions in an otherwise continuously functioning system or expose normally existing divisions masked by the functioning of a central, integrative process. In either case, dissociative states of one form or another are developed, perhaps in response to the need to retain schematic integrity or to the failure of schemas to adequately absorb a traumatic experience. Consequently, unintegrated subsystems (i.e., states or schemas) create discontinuities in experience and comprehension of experience. While these divisions are, perhaps, emotionally and schematically motivated, specific cognitive processes may be identified as the mechanisms by which these discontinuities are created and maintained. Beyond the inaccessibility of the earliest of memories due to developmental immaturities, the processes of encoding, storage, and retrieval may create disruptions in a larger parallel distributed processing network. This network of distributed memory traces, and the underlying neural networks where these traces are stored and elaborated, may be the "hardware" of schemas and dissociated states.

Considering these varied processes and multiple pathways for influence upon (and impairment of) memory for trauma, approaching psychotherapy with questions of truth or veracity of traumatic memories presents formidable challenges. Beyond questions of truth, even attempting to comprehend and understand such memory in a given individual may take considerable time and effort. Psychotherapy, in its process of creating a meaningful narrative truth for a client's life, reminds us that truth is reconstructed within the various cognitive, psychological, and neurological constraints. These constraints do not, however, preclude the truth of a client's essence, and recognizing and understanding the workings, interactions, and limitations of memory do not require that psychotherapy take on the guise of an inquisition. Indeed, the therapy relationship defines its parameters quite differently from those of legal "truth" as defined in a courtroom and allows a standard of truth quite different and significantly more complex.

However, understanding this does not implicitly suggest that all content is to be uncritically embraced and validated. Rather, an educated balance is required, necessitating a departure from the position of protecting the sanctity of the therapeutic process in respecting all content as "truth" in one sense of that word. From this position, as a profession we need to find ways to maintain a respect for both realistic appraisals of the memory process itself and the real-world implications of uncritical validation of all content brought into the therapy hour as unequivocally "true." While in most cases it is probably safe to assume that the essence of the client's truth is veridical, even if details are not, colluding with fantasied content as real, rather than understanding its meaning, does no service to a client's pursuit of growth, healing, integrity, and enhanced ability for living in a real world. Particularly with trauma, such a balance takes on significant import. As such, psychotherapists can maintain an empathic, open, respectful stance toward any client material while acknowledging the multiple layers of theory and reality in understanding memory, narrative construction, and the integration of trauma.

$$S \cdot I \cdot X$$

Traumatic Memory, Psychotherapy, and Ethics

Survivors of trauma may enter psychotherapy for any number of reasons, but often part of the work in therapy involves addressing memories of the trauma. As these memories can exist anywhere on a continuum from not knowing to vivid knowing of the trauma, therapeutic interventions should be adapted to the level of remembrance presented by the client.

Trauma Therapy as Healing

Although therapeutic processing of traumatic memories is only one element of psychotherapy with trauma survivors, it is widely thought to be an important part of the healing process. However, where suspicion of trauma exists without memory, "memory work" is contraindicated, and suggesting that healing depends on memory recovery may seriously bias the client's own natural process of growth and healing (Lindsay, 1994, 1995; Loftus, Milo, & Paddock, 1995). On the other hand, many clients come to therapy with full awareness of traumatic histories. Such a client, in directly exploring memories of trauma, is afforded the opportunity to integrate experiences that were beyond the ability of a child to endure or understand (Freud, 1917; Janet, 1892; Herman, 1992). Symptoms, feelings, and behaviors once inexplicable or ego-alien may become comprehensible to the client who can then construct a more complete and meaningful life history that includes the traumatic experience (Herman, 1992; Herman & Schatzow, 1987). Integrating memories of trauma can help the client to change irrational, destructive, or false beliefs and to develop new, adaptive survival rules (Malmo, 1990). In the process of integration, intrusive memories and dissociated ego states can be better blended into a continuous sense of self, resulting in volitional access and control of both ego states and memory (Claridge, 1992; Herman, 1992; Hyde, 1990; Janet, 1892; Spiegel et al., 1993). The recounting of childhood memories with a supportive other may allow the survivor to update childhood perceptions of and reactions to the trauma, divesting them of power. Further, the painful emotions associated with memories can be reduced and better tolerated and modulated over time (Briere, 1992; Courtois, 1991; Spiegel et al., 1993). In addition, facing such memories in adulthood can aid in removal of guilt, redirection of responsibility to other than self, and mastery of crippling fears associated with the trauma. Mastery of such fears will often enable a reduction in unmanageable and continuous physiological arousal and somatic difficulties experienced by many trauma survivors as well (Herman, 1992).

Preparation for Memory Processing

The nature of trauma can preclude easy assimilation of such events into a client's life narrative. Both at the time of the trauma and in facing memories of the experience later, survivors are faced with intense emotions, threats to basic assumptions and ways of understanding the world, and potential disintegration of ego capacities and self-structure. Further, the survivor of childhood trauma may face obstacles presented by secrecy, shame, blame, threat, and invalidation in addition to the effects of early manipulation and misrepresentation. Thus, just as the trauma itself may have been left unintegrated, later memories can be equally difficult to access in a manner that is manageable, assimilable, and therapeutic. Therefore, before focusing psychotherapy on the memory of the trauma, a solid foundation of safety, containment, and ongoing education about the process of therapy, memory, and trauma responses must be built in the therapeutic relationship as well as within the survivor.

THE THERAPEUTIC RELATIONSHIP

Before beginning therapeutic work directly with the traumatic material, a strong base of trust in the therapeutic setting must be established. The therapeutic alliance must be strong to provide psychological security, and a deeper therapeutic relationship must begin to develop in which the client senses the therapist's reliability, consistency, gentle limits, genuine caring, and sensitivity to issues of power and control (Briere, 1992; Courtois, 1991, 1992; van der Hart et al., 1989; van der Kolk & van der Hart, 1989).

For an optimal therapeutic frame with trauma survivors who have experienced massive upheaval in self and world, the therapist must be willing to move beyond neutrality in providing a holding environment in which he or she actively, calmly, and nonjudgmentally conveys safety, supportiveness, reassurance, stability, validation, and structure (Briere, 1992; Courtois, 1992; Herman, 1992; Winnicott, 1965). As with other clients, but perhaps even to a greater and more challenging degree, the therapist must be willing to assume the role of container and alter ego until the traumatized ego of the survivor can internalize these functions (McCann & Pearlman, 1990). Specifically, as the "soothing object," the therapist should be able to establish a secure bond that is taken in "and utilized to hold the psyche together when the threat of physical disintegration is reexperienced"in facing unintegrated memories (van der Kolk & Kadish, 1987, p. 188). The therapist must be able (1) to establish in the client a trust in the therapist's ability to accept, label, and hold strong emotions; (2) to structure and pace the therapy work in a manner that enhances client safety and minimizes risk of retraumatization; (3) to bear witness to the reexperience of often horrific traumatic events; (4) to maintain clear, consistent, and safe boundaries; and (5) to contain the initial chaos and fear in facing the traumatic events. Finally, the therapist should normalize and validate the client's early and current responses to known traumas and provide education about traumatic sequelae and the process of trauma work, including possible risks and benefits (Courtois, 1992; Kirschner, Kirschner, & Rappaport, 1993; Lindsay, 1995; Loftus et al., 1995).

In addition to preparation within the therapeutic relationship, the therapist may need to prepare emotionally for working directly with traumatic memories. The isolated nature of psychotherapy combined with the intensity of such memories can activate in the therapist secondary posttraumatic symptoms and countertransference reactions. These countertransference reactions may include overinvestment, distancing and avoidance, rescuing, inappropriately expressing rage, intellectualizing, or pitying, all of which may distract the client and therapist from the necessary therapy work (Briere, 1989; Courtois, 1992; Kirschner et al., 1993; McCann & Pearlman, 1990). In order to manage the intensity and attenuate such responses, the therapist's preparation for trauma work ideally will include training in working with trauma, understanding of related memory processes, and some ongoing mechanism for support and consultation (Briere, 1989).

CLIENT'S RESOURCES

In addition to focusing on the building of the therapeutic relationship in preparing for trauma work, an assessment and building of the client's psychological resources (i.e., ego strength) should be considered, particularly since trauma work can lead to, at best, an exacerbation of symptoms and, at worst, crisis and decompensation (Briere, 1989; Janet 1892; Kinston & Cohen, 1986; Kirschner et al., 1993). Particularly with traumatic experiences in early childhood, self functions may be compromised to varying degrees. In these cases, working with traumatic material must not precede therapeutic work concerned with building and strengthening self and ego functions. Specifically, evaluation of the client's readiness for trauma work would include considerations of the client's insight, intelligence, affect regulation, initiative, empathy, boundary awareness, self-soothing capacity, frustration tolerance, impulse control, and other functions involved in self-regulation (McCann & Pearlman, 1990). The specific strengths of the client should be identified and supported while he or she builds additional resources.

The initial focus should be toward fortifying ego strength. An ego strong enough to contain and integrate traumatic memories without splitting through dissociation ensures that trauma work is healing rather than retraumatizing. In psychotherapy, fortifying the ego will include helping the client (1) to gain awareness of psychological needs; (2) to strengthen an observing ego function; (3) to deepen the ability to introspect without self-blame; (4) to manage and contain increasing "doses" of emotion; (5) to tolerate being alone without loneliness; (6) to develop coping skills other than extreme dissociation or self-injury; and (7) to enhance self-soothing capacities (Courtois, 1991; Hall, 1992; McCann & Pearlman, 1990). In addition, the client should have achieved some ability for object constancy, modulation of self-loathing, capacity for self-empathy, and maintenance of psychological and physical boundaries (Hall, 1992; Hyde, 1990; McCann & Pearlman, 1990).

Further, exploration of the client's basic assumptions, beliefs, worldviews, and schemas will mark a path for the later work of assimilation, accommodation, and, eventually, integration. Both therapist and client will need to understand the basic templates of the client's life experience in order better to comprehend the areas of conflict and avoidance related to memory functioning. Such awareness may aid in predicting and possibly circumventing crises in the various phases of therapy. In addition, understanding the client's internal makeup as such will reveal openings for integration and change.

Working directly with traumatic material is contraindicated in clients who have extreme difficulty with regulation of such self functions, particularly those concerning emotional modulation, dissociative tendencies, or self-soothing (Hall, 1992). Trauma work should also be postponed and reevaluated at a later time if the client presents in a high state of arousal with intrusive images and nightmares. In such a situation, which will also likely arise periodically during the trauma work, intense unintegrated emotions, sensations, and memories of the trauma may intrude such that the client is retraumatized and his or her functioning significantly impaired. In such instances, the client should be stabilized and the intrusive phenomena contained before client and therapist commence trauma work (Herman, 1992; Horowitz, 1986; van der Hart et al., 1989; van der Kolk & van der Hart, 1989). Containment skills, ideally taught to the client in preparation for trauma work, can be utilized both in and outside of the therapy session. These techniques include the following: (1) specific safe-place imagery; (2) container imagery in which the client images a ritual for the placement of intrusive thoughts or images into a safe container; (3) grounding in which the client focuses concretely on here-and-now sensory perceptions; (4) temporary shift in therapy emphasis to here-and-now life issues, functioning, and structuring; (5) journaling; (6) adaptive use of dissociation to focus on nonthreatening material to the exclusion of the traumatic material; and (7) symbolic transformation of frightening memories through use of imagery, art, or creative writing (Briere, 1989, 1992; Courtois, 1992; Herman & Schatzow, 1987; McCann & Pearlman, 1990; Putnam, 1989; van der Hart et al., 1989; van der Hart & Friedman, 1989; van der Kolk & van der Hart, 1989). Psychotherapy techniques can be supplemented, if necessary, with medications (e.g., antidepressants, anxiolytics, etc.) in clients exhibiting high arousal or deep depression during trauma work (Courtois, 1992; van der Kolk et al., 1984; van der Kolk & Greenberg, 1987).

Memory Exploration in Psychotherapy

Addressing a client's memories for trauma in the psychotherapy setting requires considerable thought, solid clinical judgment, theoretical grounding, and awareness of ethics. As clients present with variable resources, support systems, personality dynamics, and myriad other factors, the decision to work directly with traumatic memory and the manner in which to proceed with such work require case-by-case individual assessment. In addition, the status of the client's own awareness and thinking about the trauma plays a role in such decision making. That said, however, there are general principles and issues that can be offered for use in clinical decision making about the most appropriate course of therapy with a survivor of childhood trauma.

NOT KNOWING

Clients often present for therapy with varied ways of "not knowing." For example, one client may have long-standing but vague awareness of some early trauma, and another may query the possibility of trauma given her "symptoms" of asexuality, fear of touch, depression, self-mutilation, and nightmares. Another client may have documentation of traumas for which she has no conscious memory, while still another has been informed by a former therapist that she was traumatized with neither any memory nor any prior suspicion reported by the client.

In the absence of any recognizable memory for trauma, a stance of circumspect curiosity and openness should be the rule. Although certain constellations of symptoms are quite certainly associated with trauma, these symptoms cannot be assumed to indicate conclusively the presence of trauma. Particularly when symptoms are spontaneously developed on recovery of forgotten memories, rather than present for a lifetime, the presence of early traumatization may be questionable (Terr, 1994). In any case, however, such symptoms are neither exclusive to trauma nor sufficient for any clinical judgment other than describing the current (versus historical) condition of the client and his or her functioning in the present. Terr (1994) also cautions that " 'having a feeling' about something does not make for a diagnosis" (p. 173). In other words, symptoms alone cannot be used to identify the presence or absence of distinct historical events, nor can the existence of a vague suspicion in the absence of any specific memories. Various studies have supported this position, finding that therapists have significant limitations in the ability to detect clients with repressed memories and to differentiate between accurate historical memories versus memories based on suggestion and imagination (Lindsay & Read, 1994; Enns et al., 1995). Thus it is inappropriate to suggest to a client the presence of a trauma, such as childhood sexual abuse, as an explanation for certain symptom constellations (Lindsay, 1994, 1995; Loftus et al., 1995).

Further, to assume as much and proceed with "memory work" not only defies the client's own protective mechanisms but also risks modifying whatever clarity might be present but currently inaccessible in his or her memory. Specifically, "memory work" in the absence of any definitive information about the presence or absence of trauma in a client's history can contaminate the natural progression of memory recovery if, indeed, it is adaptive for such a process to occur. As has been repeatedly established in research, memory is neither infallible nor impenetrable, and traditional forms of memory work carry the risks of distorting or interfering with the memory process. The memory system is a dynamic system in constant interaction not only with internal states and processes but also with constant input from the external world. As a result, those memories that are encoded and retained over time are elaborated, modified, schematized, and, at times, forgotten. Further, rehearsal of any content can create a "memory" for the content rehearsed. In therapy, consistently organizing the work around imaged or suspected traumatic material may possibly produce enough rehearsal to confuse the client as to the source of certain memories. Even in the absence of memories per se, a client in therapy structured around uncovering trauma may come to "believe" he or she has been traumatized and may experience the attendant crises that often occur with such realizations (Lindsay & Read, 1994; Read & Lindsay, 1994). Further, the use of invasive techniques, leading questions, or pressure to accept the therapist's hypotheses is unethical and disrespectful (Enns et al., 1995).

So, how then to proceed when suspicion of trauma arises? Nonleading exploration of the client's history, relationships, daily experiences, feelings, fears, and the like should proceed as in any psychotherapy, without use of special memory recovery techniques such as hypnosis, sodium amytal, abuse-related bibliotherapy, or use of dreams and bodily sensations as "evidence" of past events (Enns et al., 1995; Lindsay & Read, 1994). Although such symptoms may, indeed, be sequelae to trauma, to assume as much in the absence of memory is misleading. Further, using

focused techniques for memory "recovery" increases the possibility of memory distortions, enhances tendencies for dissociation, and creates a context in which the client's own process of
healing is preempted in a manner that may be overwhelming
and may lay groundwork for mistrust of that process during more
intensive and difficult phases of therapy. Such techniques also
may implicitly communicate to the client that the therapist does,
indeed, hold a special power to extract or identify a hidden
"truth," increasing the gap of power between therapist and client
and enhancing the likelihood of suggestibility.

Rather, if the client feels some vague suspicion of trauma,
this suspicion should be processed, explored, and assimilated into
the normal flow of the therapy process just as any other material
presented. In the narrative recounting of the life story, the client's
own speculations about themes and events in his or her history
inevitably arise. An exploration of the implications, meanings,
and "what-ifs" of such speculations (and their opposites) may
offer some information about the affective and schematic mo-
tives behind the client's current presentation and preoccupations
without focusing on whether or not a trauma actually occurred.
In clients presenting with notable functional amnesias (either
time-based or theme-based), generally supportive techniques
involving exploration of available memory before and after the
amnestic period and client (not therapist) speculation about life
events during the amnestic period may trigger associative networks (Horowitz, 1986; Spiegel et al., 1993). In either case, if the
client presents for therapy wondering about trauma, it is wise to
provide information and education regarding the nature of
memory for trauma and to remember that the existence of a
suspicion is no more suggestive of an actual event than are
varying symptoms (Courtois, 1991; Loftus et al., 1995; Terr,
1994).

All of this, including the provision of education to the
client, must proceed without structuring the therapy as an

archaeological dig of sorts to find a hidden trauma. At best, such a directed search might distract the therapy process from its natural direction and more salient themes. At worst, it might leave the client, perhaps unnecessarily, in confusion and crisis (Lindsay, 1994, 1995; Lindsay & Read, 1994; Loftus, 1993). Given such a suspicion, the therapist is best advised to proceed with a silent alertness to all modalities of expression, including verbal, affective, interpersonal (including transference), bodily, and sensory manifestations, as well as to remain open to other possible etiological explanations for various symptoms and dynamics (Courtois, 1992; Kinston & Cohen, 1986; Lindsay & Read, 1994). In such cases, the therapist is advised to remain aware of any internal suspicions or curiosities in attempting to prevent any implicit or explicit suggestion to the client of such biases. In the absence of current or ongoing danger or abuse, it is best left to the client to "discover" such issues in his or her life. Herman (1992) notes that "the therapist has to be reminded that she is not a fact-finder and that the reconstruction of the traumatic story is not a criminal investigation. Her role is to be an open-minded, compassionate witness, not a detective" (p. 180).

Finally, it is important to keep in mind a potential implicit message that may exist in the "not knowing" itself. A client who does not know is likely not ready to know. A respect on the part of both therapist and client for the client's own protective mechanisms and natural healing process is essential. Enns and colleagues (1995) have suggested that "loss of memory should be respected as a solution or an attempt to solve a problem because it helps clients maintain a level of psychological adjustment or equilibrium until they are ready to integrate more material into awareness" (p. 235). A sudden deluge of forgotten or long-avoided memories can overwhelm a client's defenses as well as destroy his or her sense of autonomy, empowerment, and control (Enns et al., 1995). Thus it is prudent to consider carefully the wisdom of attempting to charge through defensive layers, in recognizing that trauma, perhaps more than any other content, can catalyze crisis and decompensation in its challenges to basic schemas about self and the world (Briere, 1992; Herman, 1992). In fact, access to full memory is not necessary—and may not be possible if repeated traumas are encoded schematically—for the healing of trauma to occur (Briere, 1992; Courtois, 1992; Herman, 1992).

PARTIAL KNOWING

In the absence of a full and detailed memory of traumatic experience, partial memories may manifest themselves as disconnected fragments, highly specific body sensations, vivid perceptual experiences, unusual fight–flight–freeze responses, dreams, or intense affect shifts (Courtois, 1992). Terr (1994) notes that partial representations such as these often have manifested as lifelong, often incomprehensible, patterns in those with actual traumatic memories (versus individuals presenting with or recovering potentially illusory memories that may produce symptoms not previously apparent in the behavioral repertoire). With such memory fragments, the therapist is advised to proceed only with that material that has achieved conscious, verbal, comprehensible representation. As the nonverbal symptoms may be either very direct expressions of early trauma or symptoms with other etiologies, to validate these as veridical memories carries considerable risk. However, even with verbal memories, very careful trauma work can proceed if, and only if, the client expresses a clear desire and readiness to do such work.

If the client expresses ambivalence, it may be first most appropriate to explore this ambivalence. This exploration might include consideration of the meaning of knowing versus the meaning of not knowing, the worst fears and fantasied results of exploring, safety needs and concerns, and other concerns of daily functioning (Claridge, 1992). Further, it may be that in the proposed hierarchical organization of memory into schematic matrices or networks, access to higher-level memories or issues may first require working through nested sets of interdependent lower-level memories or issues (e.g., establishing safety parameters as noted above, securing supportive relationships, identifying and remediating skill deficits) (Bruhn, 1990; Neisser, 1986).

Direct work with partial memory should be embedded in a general exploration of other events and circumstances in the client's past and current life. This creates a continuous narrative context within which to place the memories without reinforcement of the isolation, encapsulation, or dissociation of traumatic material (Herman, 1992). Within this context, the *available* memory fragments, along with the client's reactions to these memories, can be explored, rather than focusing exclusively on the excavation of unavailable memories (Herman, 1992; McCann & Pearlman, 1990). It may be helpful to remember that information encoded in nonverbal modalities may be "less accessible, sometimes less comprehensible, and often less communicable" (Bonanno, 1990b, p. 183). However, since traumatic memory may be, in part, state-dependent, specific cues or emotional states activated in working with existing memory may, in fact, stimulate association (Bruhn, 1990; Courtois, 1992; Levis, 1990). Such associations may then be explored through a nondirective examination of sensory, motoric, and verbal details and associations, with the goal of gradual representation in conceptual–verbal modes that allow greater conscious awareness and understanding (Bonanno, 1990a). Additionally, identifying cues to arousal as well as patterns of arousal also may be an aid in understanding observed associative linking (Briere, 1992; Claridge, 1992; Levis, 1990). Briere (1992) believes that memory exploration needs no further "technique" or direction, as gentle, nonintrusive trauma work will slowly move the client into affective and cognitive experiences that allow gradual access to

state-dependent material. He believes that safety and trust between client and therapist are the only prerequisites to memory
retrieval and cautions that shortcuts generally are not helpful.

Others, however, allow a slightly more active, but still
nondirective and nonintrusive, exploration. Along these lines,
representation of the *available* memory fragments through nondirective imaging (e.g., "When you're ready an image will come
to mind that will help you get where you need to go in your
healing journey") can be used to stimulate nonverbal, less
conscious modalities during the session (Hyde, 1990, p. 175). This
technique also can be used in focusing on the body and imaging
(nondirectively) whatever comes to mind in relation to feelings
or tension experienced somatically (Hyde, 1990; Turner, 1990).
Or, development of metaphors, production of art (e.g., drawing,
clay), use of journals, dream work, and enactive exercises (e.g.,
Gestalt empty chair) may enhance the expression, translation,
and organization of verbal and contextual information only
weakly associated due to selective inattention or poor elaboration. Such techniques may stimulate mature verbal insight by
concrete visual representation of the internal environment
(Courtois, 1992; Greenberg & van der Kolk, 1987; van der Hart
et al., 1989). Further, these techniques are ambiguous enough to
enable a safe emotional distance for gradual comprehension of
nonverbal material (Bonanno, 1990a; Briere, 1989; Claridge,
1992; Greenberg & van der Kolk, 1987; Kirschner et al., 1993;
Weiser, 1990).

Again, however, it is important that such therapeutic interventions avoid the context of a search for hidden trauma but,
rather, take the form of an exploration of what currently is
available. As such, it is imperative to avoid any form of repeated
or coercive questioning of the client, as repeated questioning
can, over time, serve as a form of rehearsal that results in deep
encoding of related images and thoughts, eventually creating
"memories" that may be indistinguishable from memories for

actual historical events (Ceci & Bruck, 1993). Further along these lines, the inquiries that the therapist does make should be matter-of-fact and nonleading. Particularly at this stage of knowing, clients often are in need of validation and affirmation of their memories and the meaning of such memories. In this situation, resisting the pull to confirm requires considerable ability in the therapist to tolerate the attendant uncertainty and anxiety of the client (Ceci & Bruck, 1993).

FULL KNOWING

Many, if not most, survivors of childhood trauma consciously know, and have always known, about their traumatic experiences. In some cases, the "knowing" even takes the form of eidetic, highly specific, and detailed memories that are intrusive and even terrifying to the client. Unlike clients with no memories or only partial memories who often are obsessed to search, clients who do have memories sometimes wish that they did not and actively attempt to suppress, withhold, or deny their experiences (Briere, 1992; Courtois, 1992; Herman & Schatzow, 1987). And if psychological defenses do not mute the memories, often somatization, drug use, high-risk behaviors, or transient psychotic episodes will (Herman & Schatzow, 1987). In these cases, trauma work cannot proceed until such symptoms are relieved and better coping mechanisms developed (Courtois, 1991).

Even with full knowing, integration may be incomplete, with a side-by-side existence of "normal" history and trauma history. The thought of integration of the trauma may produce intensely painful emotions in addition to fears of losing control, loss of important relationships, or judgment of others (Briere, 1992; Herman & Schatzow, 1987). Here especially careful examination of schemas about self and world in addition to basic assumptions and salient needs will be necessary for integration of the traumatic memories.

INTEGRATION

Therapists working with traumatic memory are reminded that the goal is "integration—not exorcism," implying that effective psychotherapy work with traumatic memory will promote not abreaction and catharsis but rather gradual mastery, integration, and understanding (Enns et al., 1995; Herman, 1992, p. 181; McCann & Pearlman, 1990). Thus the goal is not expressing the memories per se but, rather, discerning the meaning and place of such memories in the whole of a client's life. In fact, Herman (1992) suggests that trauma work that fails in "providing an adequate context for integration [is] therapeutically irresponsible and potentially dangerous, for [it leaves] the patient without the resources to cope with the memories uncovered" (p. 184). In addition, Horowitz (1986) notes that in psychotherapy with trauma survivors and their memories:

> Consciousness for the sake of awareness alone is not the goal; rather, conscious contemplation is used as a tool for unlearning automatic associations and resolving seemingly irreconcilable conflicts. Change is accomplished by a combination of conscious and unconscious processes, by the revisions, learning, and the creation of new solutions required by the altered situation. In other words, change can be explained as decisions, both conscious and unconscious, that revise inner schemata and plans for action. The goal is continuity of the traumatic experience with other life memories. (p. 99)

Thus full integration is possible only as information encoded in all modalities is translated into verbal representation, transformed into acceptable, assimilable forms, and placed in the life narrative (Bonanno, 1990b; Herman, 1992; Horowitz, 1986; Malmo, 1990; Spiegel et al., 1993).

With a prior understanding of the client's adult schemas, needs, and assumptions, the therapist can slowly work with traumatic images to change the accompanying frozen, childlike, and often inaccurate beliefs, enabling greater correspondence with adult beliefs (Malmo, 1990). As the memories, emotions, and cognitions of the traumatized child are integrated within the frame of adult interpretation and understanding, old perceptions are updated. For example, the client may understand for the first time that her own reactions during the trauma indicated helplessness rather than immorality. Moreover, this integration can encourage forgiveness of self and desensitize the client to early, primitive emotions that were intolerable to an undeveloped ego structure (Briere, 1992; Herman, 1992; McCann & Pearlman, 1990; van der Hart et al., 1989; van der Kolk & van der Hart, 1989; Weiser, 1990). This process will necessitate provision of a frame or scaffolding by the therapist to help the client organize, label, categorize, and express the traumatic experience until, gradually, he or she can accomplish these functions for himself or herself. The result of such processes should be the working through and incorporation of traumatic material into revised schemas and a more fully developed life narrative (Horowitz, 1986).

Throughout the course of trauma work, integration can be encouraged by allowing memories to occur while gently interfering with reflexive dissociation or other cognitive controls or defenses in the client (Briere, 1992; Horowitz, 1986). This allows the client to bring memories and responses to the trauma into a safe, healing, and empowered context that will allow reformulation of the trauma's meaning. The interruption of dissociative processes in the therapy hour also supports the client's development of capacities for maintaining conscious awareness while accessing the traumatic material in a context of safe containment. In this setting, clients can learn that strong feelings are not invariably associated with the occurrence of trauma (Briere, 1992). Over time as memories are repeatedly invoked in a safe environment, the traumatic memories will be paired instead with the safety and containment of the therapeutic environment which, eventually, will be internalized by the client. Further, the intense emotions, if elicited with careful pacing and ongoing integration, can be validated, supported, and normalized leading to increased emotional tolerance and modulation over time (Briere, 1992; Claridge, 1992; McCann & Pearlman, 1990; Spiegel et al., 1993).

When working directly with the traumatic material, a balance of exploration and containment are required in order for effective integration to occur. At any phase of memory exploration, the psyche's own regulatory mechanisms may allow existing or new memories to intrude into awareness, adaptively shut down before becoming overwhelming, and continually return until their impact is absorbed gradually (Horowitz, 1986). The absorption will reflect a self-regulatory balance between the accommodation of schemas to contain new information and the assimilation of the information with some modification allowing minimal disruption to schemas (Claridge, 1992; Herman, 1992; Horowitz, 1986). Although much of this process of pacing and control will be in the hands of the client, the therapist may intervene to slow the process in the event that the client becomes overwhelmed. Pacing can be thought of as a kind of "dosing" procedure where the therapist balances trauma work with supportive work, allowing gradual integration that permits the client to metabolize small bits of the trauma and adapt at each step of the process (Claridge, 1992; Horowitz, 1986; Kirschner et al., 1993; McCann & Pearlman, 1990; Spiegel et al., 1993; van der Kolk & Kadish, 1987).

During this process, the therapist must retain a global focus on the whole of the client's current life and history in order to avoid colluding in the encapsulation and amplification of the traumatic material. In some clients with long histories of trauma, particularly interpersonal trauma, a diffuse identity can be replaced by an "abuse identity" that perpetuates the identification of the abuse as the primary feature in the client's life, repeating in a distorted manner the primacy of the perpetrator in earlier life. Thus, continued work with the client's current issues, functioning, work, relationships, and leisure activities can support pacing and reinforce integration into the current and historical life narrative. This allows consideration of implications of the traumatic experience in terms of the present and the future and can aid in the avoidance of a sense of being consumed by the trauma. In this way, the trauma is no longer a primary, magnified presence in the survivor's life but, instead, becomes integrated with other negative and positive life experiences in supporting a balanced and unified sense of self. Harvey and Herman (1994) cogently summarize the nature of trauma work in psychotherapy, noting:

> Contrary to the portrait of clinical work with trauma survivors being promulgated by the popular press and the false memory literature, the aim of clinical exploration of the traumatic past is neither to uncover more and more horror, nor to assign blame and responsibility for adult life to others, but rather to help the adult survivor name and assign meaning and comprehensibility to the past, to facilitate the integration of traumatic remembrance into an ongoing personal narrative, and to help the patient grieve the past and be freed of it. (p. 304)

The Question of Truth Revisited

The question of truth considered in more intellectual, philosophical realms exists on a level of abstraction somewhat removed from the intensity and intimacy of the therapy relationship. The extraordinary pain and uncertainty of the individual client in the presence of an empathic therapist magnifies the importance of this issue. With the lack of integration of most traumatic material, the client has a compulsion to know and to integrate as well as a drive to deny and forget. Further, clients who have been traumatized, particularly those who have experienced repeated traumas, may harbor serious doubts and insecurities about their own perceptions and beliefs. In the intensity of the therapy work where the traumatic material is being directly faced, this conflict may be particularly prominent. The pull for the therapist not only to "know" the truth with certainty but to validate the client's perceptions of this truth can be powerful.

If we assume, in general, that one of the tasks of therapy is to articulate a continuous life narrative that may or may not be unequivocally accurate in the sense of an objective, historical truth (if there is, indeed, an objective truth), then the question of veracity seems less relevant. The essential factor really becomes the mastery of whatever is uncovered, with little or no contamination from therapist bias (Ganaway, 1991b). Although historical veridicality and detailed accuracy are necessary in a courtroom setting, it is essential that we refrain from courtroom conduct and standards in the psychotherapy setting. Such a shift would have dramatic implications in the most basic ways we interact with and understand our clients.

However, in working with traumatic memory, clients often express strong desires for validation. Uncritically validating any and all memories, given the extraordinary intrapsychic and relational consequences of discovering trauma, may encourage in the client lax decision criteria in evaluating the source and reality of retrieved memories, increasing the chance of suggestibility. In addition, before a client is supported in organizing therapy or basing life decisions on such memories, it may be helpful to consider in therapy the possibility of both verification and falsification and what either would mean to the client (Terr, 1994). Further, if the therapist takes the responsibility for believing or disbelieving from the client, the client's ambivalence is embodied in a way that can create polarization between therapist and client. This polarization may allow the client to adhere fully to one side or the other without resolving the conflict internally in a manner that encourages self-validation and self-trust. Ganaway (1989) notes that "the patient ultimately must reinternalize the insatiable need for external validation . . . in order to work through the mistrust of her own perceptions and memories until finally reaching a level of self-validation that will give her a sense of mastery over what once was a fragmented internal world of interwoven fact, fantasy, and illusion" (p. 216). This allows fuller experience of the original rage, betrayal, disappointment, and pain, all of which are necessary if the traumatic experience is to be made fully conscious and integrated. This also allows the client to come to terms with his or her own final truth that will emerge over time through integration (Ganaway, 1989, 1991b; Lindsay, 1995).

Ethical Considerations

As with most applied clinical situations, psychotherapy with trauma survivors, particularly in regard to trauma work, requires much consideration of ethical issues. Specifically, since much trauma involves interpersonal threat and boundary violation, the therapy setting with its intensity, isolation, and intimacy creates potential for great difficulty if not conducted within a frame of utmost professionalism and integrity.

Maintaining such a frame first requires the therapist to consider the boundaries of competence in terms of training and preparation to engage in trauma work with trauma survivors (American Psychological Association, 1992). The therapist working with the trauma survivor should have training in the sequelae and dynamics of trauma as well as the specifics of trauma work, containment, possible symptom exacerbation, and related crisis resolution. Education in related areas of cognitive processing and memory functioning will also guide the therapist in this work. In fact, any work with traumatic memory may demand that the therapist be at least acquainted with the relevant cognitive theory and research and with the risks associated with traditional forms of memory work (e.g., hypnosis, sodium amytal). And with this education, the therapist should practice only within the framework of what is known about memory, its fallibility, and the relationship of symptoms to trauma and memory. While therapists are trained to interpret, help organize thoughts and emotions, increase insight and understanding, and other functions, the training does not prepare one to "read" the patient's past or predict the future. Clear awareness of this distinction and a commitment to think critically about the process of psychotherapy with trauma and its underlying theoretical bases are essential aspects of competent practice.

Given both the apparent prevalence of childhood trauma and the demands and uncertainty of working with traumatic memory, it is essential for the therapist also to consider personal problems or conflicts in relation to this work. Basic issues such as therapist needs, biases, values, beliefs, and limitations must be considered relative to the impact on work with trauma and traumatic memory (Enns et al., 1995). The therapist who has a history of trauma may find such work particularly challenging in terms of overidentification, projection, boundary confusion, and stimulation of trauma-related images and emotions (Briere, 1989; Kirschner et al., 1993). This will be particularly difficult for the therapist who has not yet achieved integration or a sense of resolution in the healing process. Even the therapist without a trauma history may find personal problems interfering with the energy required for such work or developing in response to the work. The potential for countertransferential acting out in any of these situations requires the therapist to consider carefully the demands of working with trauma survivors and to obtain psychotherapy or, at minimum, ongoing peer support and consultation (American Psychological Association, 1992; Briere, 1989; Enns et al., 1995).

Related to both competence and personal capability are issues concerning the safety and avoidance of harm to the client. An absolute given is a prohibition of any form of sexual intimacy with a client. Although this applies with equal force to any client–therapist dyad, trauma survivors are especially at risk for harm in this way. Particularly since trauma can render the survivor prone to freezing responses, passivity, and helplessness in the face of danger or threat, these clients may require special sensitivity and awareness of boundaries on the part of the therapist. This sensitivity must also extend to issues of dual relationships and contact outside the therapy session, since trauma survivors often request and sometimes need support beyond once-a-week therapy sessions. Sensitivity to boundaries and minimization of confusion for the client will require the ability in the therapist to set clear, gentle limits to avoid ambiguity in the relationship (American Psychological Association, 1992).

Also related to avoiding harm to the client is the potential for misuse of the therapist's power. In the Ethical Principles of Psychologists, the section on "Concern for Others' Welfare" (Principle E) (American Psychological Association, 1992, p. 1600) notes that psychologists must be "sensitive to real and ascribed differences in power between themselves and others, and they do not exploit or mislead other people during or after professional relationships" (p. 1600). The client is often biased to rely on the therapist for identifying some "truth" in his or her life, as the therapist is often seen as the credible authority (Ceci & Bruck, 1993). Particularly with trauma survivors who may have a propensity for dissociative reactions and spontaneous age regression back to split-off or "frozen" parts of self, this power differential can become even more pronounced. In addition, given the uncertainty of the trauma work and the frequent lack of self-trust in trauma clients, the need for validation can place a great deal of power in the therapist's hands. The therapist must take great care not to create an "atmosphere of accusation" in which the therapist perceives himself or herself as holding or sharing the client's awareness and rage concerning a hidden trauma (Ceci & Bruck, 1993, p. 421). Such a stance, implicit or explicit, can set the stage for a coercive atmosphere in which the client feels compelled to respond. The therapist must be sensitive to this issue in continually affirming the dignity of the client and in maintaining the fine balance between necessary support and respectful empowerment of the client throughout the therapy work (Herman, 1992; Janet, 1892).

Particularly concerning the validation of traumatic memories, the therapist must be aware of the potential of his or her influence on this work. Certainly the therapist should never conclusively inform the client that trauma has occurred, even if the therapist suspects as much. It is also most ethical to avoid assumptions and interpretations about the facts or meanings of traumatic events. For example, to infer or suggest rage in a client who has been abused may create internal conflict in the client who is not feeling rage at all. Further, to assume rage and organize therapeutic interventions accordingly may preempt the client's need and responsibility to develop and hold such feelings in himself or herself. Such interpretations can be neither entirely objective nor effectively untangled from the therapist's own theoretical biases, personal experiences, emotional reactions, needs, beliefs, and values. As such, and particularly with the import and impact of trauma, no suggestion should be made in this regard to a client given the impact of the therapist's power in the reconstruction of the client's life narrative, particularly with ambiguous and potentially frightening historical content (American Psychological Association, 1992; Courtois, 1992; Ganaway, 1989; Herman, 1992; Kirschner, 1993; Loftus, 1993; McCann & Pearlman, 1990; Morris, 1993; Pynoos & Nader, 1989; Spence, 1982).

In this regard, Eth (1988) offers very specific guides for ethical trauma work, including suggestions never to: ask leading or suggestive questions; cue, reinforce, or encourage compliance in producing memories; reward elaborations or embellishments; introduce details of the traumas of others into the client's narrative; or provide provocative or stimulating materials to trigger memories. In the same spirit, Loftus (1993) cautions therapists never to "probe relentlessly for recalcitrant memories," as "zealous conviction is a dangerous substitute for an open mind" (p. 534). In considering the impact of the therapist's power in the therapy setting, she considers the possibility that such dynamics in the therapist can lead to fixed beliefs that may precipitate decompensation in the client. She suggests instead using "clarification, compassion, and gentle confrontation along with a demonstration of empathy for the painful struggles these patients must endure as they come to terms with their personal truths" (Loftus, 1993, p. 534).

Finally, the consideration of the influence of psychotherapists, particularly psychologists, in sociopolitical realms must never be underestimated. Given the current controversy surrounding issues of early memory and trauma, the profession must be cognizant of the need to become educated and informed on this issue. As scientists and practitioners, we must be willing to ask difficult questions of our own personal, theoretical, and political belief systems in considering the impact of these issues on our lives, the lives of our clients and their families, and on social acceptance or denial of trauma. In considering that the questions we now ask were asked of Freud a century ago, we may see the vicissitudes of social opinion and power distribution from a cyclical historical context that suggests the real issue lies less in the "truth" of traumatic memory than in the sociocultural reaction to such truths. The reality of trauma, particularly childhood trauma involving forms of interpersonal abuse, is difficult to face in that it threatens many schemas within the collective psyche. We must ask ourselves why we find it necessary as a social system and as a profession to demand a higher standard of proof for traumatic material than any other content that a client brings into the therapy session. Briere (1992) states this dilemma in regard to trauma by noting:

> The therapist must question herself as to why the "real facts" are so important. . . . In other areas of psychotherapy, it is often benignly assumed that clients' reports of past events—although frequently distorted by defenses and previous experiences—are essentially true, and the client is rarely cross-examined as to the detailed aspects of her historical account. . . . It is in this regard that the clinician must examine his or her assumptions: Do I especially question the honesty of this disclosure in part because I have been trained (socially and professionally) to doubt reports of . . . victimization? To the extent that this answer is affirmative, resolution of the veracity question may ultimately become a therapist's (as opposed to client's) issue. (pp. 53–54)

We must consider such issues in terms of the role of our profession in the legal and legislative systems, and we must consider the conflict in those roles with our responsibilities to our clients' best interests and to ourselves. Given the very different standard—and even meaning—of truth between the courtroom and the psychotherapy setting, we must question our own belief systems about each of these and their relative importance as well as our roles in either encouraging, remaining uninvolved, or discouraging clients seeking litigation related to early traumas. To what extent does such involvement in litigation keep the client in a traumatized and invalidated position in which he or she continues to have life dominated by trauma? To what extent does not seeking retribution affect the empowerment of the individual?

And related to all of this, we must consider the impact of our public statements, or the lack thereof, in regard to a potentially harmful controversy that is sweeping our culture. As a profession, and as individuals representing this profession, it is important to seek out education and information in order to speak intelligently, clearly, and even dispassionately in a way that ensures the integrity and rights of our profession and our clients. It is important that we not become organized by a polarized sociocultural debate that may have as much to do with real issues concerning false allegations as with collective denial of the darker truths of humanity. It is incumbent upon our profession to clarify these issues, first within scientific realms, and then in more public arenas, rather than to support one side of a battle that no one can win. As such, in bringing scientific and clinical knowledge into courtroom or media settings, it may be helpful to explore and understand our own internal biases and agendas, as well as to ensure the ability of our profession to see various facets of these issues and to represent the "truth" as scientifically and clinically validated to the best of our abilities.

Research Considerations

In considering research on memory for traumatic experience, we must question certain epistemological and related paradigmatic assumptions. The prevailing scientific epistemology most often assumes the primacy of empirical or experimental verification in validating the existence of a phenomenon. Indeed, the rigor and clarity of empirical science, along with the contributions of experimental paradigms in the understanding of psychological phenomena, ensure a significant place for empiricism and the experimental method in the repertoire of scientific exploration. However, other ways of "knowing" exist, and particularly in regard to complex human processes, it is important to consider the nature of the questions we ask, the implications of the methods we use to answer those questions, and the ways these questions as well as our belief systems influence outcomes, inferences, and generalizations. Erdelyi and Goldberg (1979) have noted that

> methodology, after all, is only an applied epistemology; as such it is a band of philosophy and, therefore, theory; as such it is subject to verification—and, hopefully, to falsification. If an applied epistemological theory fails, it should be discarded or modified, like any theory. There is nothing

sacrosanct or final about theories, whether about the mind (psychological theory) or about how the mind should pursue truth (methodological theories). (p. 384)

In regard to complex phenomena such as repression, these authors believe that experimental theories have fallen short, and they query "since when, and . . . by what philosophy of science, is a phenomenon's existence predicated on the laboratory scientist's ability to create it?" (Erdelyi & Goldberg, 1979, p. 359). Indeed, even Freud observed that other paradigms were valid, at least in clinical settings, for understanding complex phenomena. Erdelyi and Goldberg (1979) note that Freud viewed "with alternate bemusement and incredulity the insistence of experimental psychologists to foist the ceremonial rigors of the laboratory upon the obvious" (p. 367).

The rational epistemology, as described by MacKay (1988), rejects assumptions that tightly controlled and isolated empirical findings can be directly applicable to complex, multiply determined psychological phenomena. Pervin (1990) concurs, noting, "not only may there be multiple determinants of a phenomenon, but the same phenomenon can be caused by different sets of determinants. Thus, in understanding phenomena we may discover many causes, all of which are potentially relevant but no one of which is necessary or sufficient" (p. 724). The rational epistemology suggests that real-world phenomena require creative, complex solutions that are theory driven, rather than data driven as are the findings of more reductionistic methods of science. This epistemology would agree with Erdelyi and Goldberg (1979) who caution researchers about tendencies for "shaping reality to fit the method" (p. 384). In fact, it may be that "social entities, as unique historical products, can only be *interpreted* or *understood*" because with humans, the falsification premise of science is not always possible (Kirschner, 1993, p. 220). Indeed, fuller understanding is required if we are to interpret the findings of experimental studies which, by necessity, assume that understanding of the parts will inherently lead to understanding of the whole.

For example, much research and meta-analysis has been conducted to investigate the various "parts" of the phenomenon of repression, with the conclusion in some quarters that repression does not exist and, therefore, "recovered" memories are suspect (e.g., Holmes, 1990; Loftus, 1993). What is missing here is the *fact* that traumatic forgetting does, without dispute, occur. Open for debate are the cognitive and dynamic mechanisms underlying such forgetting, as well as the related motivations or purposes. Repression may, indeed, be a less parsimonious explanation; however, that fact does not negate the existence of the phenomenon. Careful thought and a fuller sense of understanding might suggest that the question here is one of semantics more than one of science. Thus in studying human behavior and psychological processes, it is imperative that we refuse myopia, opting at times instead for less precise but perhaps more complex and sophisticated ways of understanding and interpreting.

Memory Research

Historically, most memory research in cognitive science has consisted of well-controlled laboratory studies. However, increasing attention is being directed to the ecological validity of such studies in understanding the actual functioning of human memory in real-life situations (Erdelyi, 1990; Erdelyi & Goldberg, 1979; Goodman et al., 1990; Kirschner, 1993; MacKay, 1988; Neisser, 1988; van der Kolk & van der Hart, 1991). Schachtel (1947, 1959) seemed to foresee this dilemma in the following observation:

> Obviously the concept of memory . . . cannot be the impersonal, artificial, isolated, and abstract concept implied by

experimentation on the recall of digits, nonsense syllables, and similar material, a concept which seems more appropriate for the testing of the capacity of some mechanical apparatus than for the understanding of the functioning of memory in the living person. . . . Nobody doubts that it is easier to remember meaningful than meaningless material and that the function of memory has not developed in order to make possible the recall of nonsense. Memory as a function of the living personality can be understood only as a capacity for the organization and reconstruction of past experiences and impressions in the service of present needs, fears, and interests. It goes without saying that just as there is no such thing as impersonal perception and impersonal experience, there is also no impersonal memory. (1947, p. 191)

Others note specific problems in much of the current memory research. Some of these include the lack of clinical input and applicability of much memory research; the lack of attention to functional disorders of memory; the use of nonengaging, uninteresting, mundane events usually involving bystanders (versus participants); and the querying of peripheral rather than central details. It is speculated that the result of such research misrepresents complex human abilities for accurate, real-life event recall (Erdelyi, 1990; Erdelyi & Goldberg, 1979; Goodman et al., 1990; van der Kolk & van der Hart, 1991). Further, others have suggested that empirical findings on normal populations cannot be assumed to generalize to traumatized populations without research comparing the two (Courtois, 1995).

In general, it may be that the lack of relevant research in the area of trauma and memory is attributable to inadequate research methods and paradigms (Goodman et al., 1994). Further, in the polarization of this issue, domains have been crossed, perhaps unfruitfully, with cognitive researchers focused on the critique of clinical practice and clinicians focused on the critique of cognitive paradigms and observations. In both cases, there likely exists some lack of familiarity with the crossed domain. Thus rather than further polarizing this debate by criticizing the "opponent's" domain, perhaps both clinicians and cognitive scientists might better combine their strengths and considerable knowledge bases to promote understanding by all concerned parties (Berliner & Williams, 1994; Courtois, 1995).

The nature of trauma poses particular problems for memory research. Specifically, and simply, trauma cannot be created in a controlled, laboratory setting. Experimental paradigms that purport generalizability to real-life trauma rely on the induction of stress or unpleasant feelings, which do not approximate the intensity or threat of direct experience of trauma. Further, the focus (and findings) of much of this research is on peripheral details rather than essence. While such details are, in fact, important in the courtroom, in clinical work with trauma, the crucial factor is the essence of the traumatic event and its meaning to the client. If we applied narrow laboratory analogue findings to clinical settings, we might find ourselves judging and doubting each utterance of our clients, requiring corroboration and proof to the exclusion of deeper, more complex understandings. To understand the nature of the interaction between trauma and memory functioning, it is essential to consider alternative epistemologies and more ecologically valid paradigms for research.

In developing ecologically valid research, striving to approximate the elegance of the controlled, clear methodology of experimental research is ideal. However, in aiming for a sophisticated understanding of memory processes, it may be that we sacrifice some of this elegance in the spirit of capturing the essence of the functioning of memory in trauma survivors. Field research (such as that conducted by Terr), clinical observations (e.g., Janet, Freud, Herman), exploratory research, and phenomenological study conducted retrospectively with survivors of real-life trauma may yield greater understanding of this phenomenon than that afforded by strictly controlled laboratory paradigms. For example, Loftus and her colleagues (Loftus, 1979, 1993; Loftus & Loftus, 1980; Loftus & Christianson, 1989; Loftus et al., 1992) have made influential generalizations about clinical manifestations of traumatic memory based on laboratory studies of induced stress and subsequent recall of details. It is not clear that all of the clinical inferences concerning traumatic memory are warranted based on this research (Berliner & Williams, 1994). While this research does offer important information about the nature of memory as it functions in specific settings, it may be important to remember the multiple determinations and complexity of such phenomena in making only conservative inferences and generalizations concerning the applicability of these findings to actual trauma. In fact, Terr (1994) has noted that laboratory-based analogue studies, often conducted using university students, do not apply well "to the perception, storage, and retrieval of such things as childhood murders, rapes, or kidnappings" (p. 51). She continues by suggesting that "experiments on college students do not simulate clinical instances of trauma. And they have little to do with childhood itself" (p. 52).

Further, the social, cultural, and familial pressures around trauma, particularly interpersonal trauma, impose significant factors to be accounted for in understanding trauma and memory, factors that cannot be replicated in laboratory or analogue studies. Thinking critically about such issues is an intrinsic part of the social scientist's training. However, such thinking should not prevent openness to the ideas in this body of work that are, in fact, quite helpful to the clinician seriously committed to a fuller understanding of the research and theoretical issues surrounding traumatic memory.

Perhaps more valid for understanding more complex clinical manifestations of traumatic memory are the studies conducted by Terr (1983, 1988, 1990, 1991). Her studies involve systematic and well-documented investigation of children who have survived verified traumatic events. In longitudinal follow-up over many years, Terr's field research allows exploration of the performance of memory for trauma over the course of development and maturation, life changes, and normally interfering factors (e.g., discussions with significant others, news reports, etc.) in naturalistic settings. While her methodology has been criticized for leaving many factors uncontrolled and thus unable to be accounted for in explaining her observations, analogue research may be similarly criticized for excluding key factors, limiting application and generalizability. Terr's research does offer ecological validity in demonstrating memory performance in interaction with the very real limitations and interferences of life as it is lived. However, since neither paradigm seems sufficient, the optimal solution may be to reach for synthesis.

Indeed, as Briere (1995) points out, most current approaches are imperfect. Analogue studies suffer limits in generalizability, whereas field studies are limited by the difficulty in corroboration and clarity of interpretation of results. However, Pervin (1990) optimistically observes that current research increasingly uses field methodologies that are more programmatic in nature and less firmly tied to specific questionnaires or tests. He, and others (e.g., Erdelyi & Goldberg, 1979; MacKay, 1988), anticipate technological and methodological advances that will allow the ability to conduct such research with even greater precision and elegance as that afforded by experimental paradigms. The realm of ecological memory research, as represented by Neisser (1988), has laid the groundwork for rapprochement in this regard. Other cognitive scientists (Erdelyi, 1990), and certainly other disciplines (such as anthropology), have worked to systematize exploratory, observational, and field methodologies with much success. Particularly those proponents of ecological approaches to memory research are achieving a rapprochement between the rigor of the laboratory and the realism of naturalistic settings (Neisser, 1988; Winograd, 1988). Perhaps both clinicians and cognitive scientists increasingly can work together to combine the strength of each realm in finding both complex and precise ways to understand traumatic memory.

Questions for Future Study

The interaction of trauma with memory is an area rich for exploration. However, the questions of interest vary relative to the many issues evoked by consideration of trauma and memory. Specifically, Harvey and Herman (1994) suggest that research might be divided into three realms of study. The first is forensic in nature and is devoted to issues of "truth" relative to due process and the weight of evidence in testimony. The second concerns clinical practice with trauma or suspected trauma. And the third set of issues is focused on memory research per se, concerning issues such as the role of strong emotion in encoding, storage, and retrieval, the nature of traumatic memories, and the process of memory impairment for trauma. The following discussion of research centers primarily on clinical concerns, with an eye toward the collaboration of cognitive scientists and clinicians in understanding the complex phenomenon of traumatic memory.

One area of inquiry is the natural progression of memory after traumatic events that are experienced individually or in groups. Longitudinal field studies of survivors of traumatic events may provide descriptive detail about the nature of traumatic memory. In particular, disasters provide opportunities for such research both in the immediate and long-term traumatic memory functioning. Increasing clarification of questions and methods of inquiry in such field studies will strengthen this base of knowledge. Similarly, longitudinal studies following documented trauma in individual children (perhaps through emergency room records) may shed light on the natural functioning of memory for individually experienced traumatic events. It would be interesting to explore the differences in memory functioning for shared traumatic experiences in groups (e.g., natural disasters) versus individual traumas (e.g., sexual abuse).

Another line of inquiry might involve the nature of the interaction between long-term memory for childhood trauma and the process of clarifying a life narrative in psychotherapy. Perhaps the initial question should concern outcome research concerning the necessity of memory work in therapy. Specifically, to query whether or not retrieval of traumatic memories provides, in itself, therapeutic benefit is paramount to clinical work with trauma. If such work is determined to be therapeutic, then a consideration of specific client dynamics for such memory work as particularly useful or contraindicated is essential. Further, a determination of beneficial versus risky techniques for trauma work could serve as a guide to clinicians working with individuals with suspected trauma histories (Harvey & Herman, 1994; Lindsay, 1995).

In addition, psychotherapy process research in this area might consider the influence of the schemas and belief systems of both therapists and clients on the process and outcome of psychotherapy. Process and outcome effects related to the therapists' own history of trauma would be interesting to explore. Horowitz (1986, 1988, 1991) and others have developed sound coding methodologies for clarifying schematic biases in process research. Such research could be conducted using actual psychotherapy sessions, or a more controlled method might use one to two psychotherapy interviews conducted by real therapists blind to a trained research confederate "client." In addition, it might be possible to elucidate the therapeutic process further by providing immediately to both therapist and client a transcript of the session onto which each could note internal thoughts, assumptions, interpretations, and feelings that occurred during, and perhaps influenced the direction of, the session.

In looking at the natural progression of traumatic memory recovery and integration, an exploratory study might code interventions and responses over the longer-term course of traumatic memory work over time in psychotherapy. In this regard, group therapy settings, in both inpatient and outpatient settings, might also be studied for differences in directive versus nondirective therapy styles and influence of the narratives of other group members on the content and processing of an individual's memorial and narrative reconstruction. Process coding could be used in such a study in addition to outcome variables concerning self-development, integration, dissociative tendencies, schematic change, and memory functioning.

Finally, an ongoing project of mine involves the exploration of the relationship between self-development and autobiographical memory as related to trauma. As memory impairment in trauma has been speculated to relate to self-impairment (i.e., in the form of schemas, ego strength, sense of self, integration, etc.), and since self-impairment is theoretically thought to result from early trauma, it is of interest to study the interaction of self, memory, and trauma. Several autobiographical memory paradigms offer methods to study retrospectively the nature of memory for trauma, and various tools for exploring self-development exist. These methods, in conjunction with structured clinical interviews and/or questionnaires concerning dissociative tendencies, may reveal interesting and applicable interactions between traumatic memory and self-impairment that are currently only theoretically or anecdotally described in the literature.

Summary: Traumatic Memory Research

The area of memory for trauma represents a rich and open realm for further exploration through research. Few systematic studies have adequately captured the essence of traumatic memory; thus much is needed in order to understand this phenomenon and its clinical implications. Given the significant impact on the lives of individuals in psychotherapy, it is essential that researchers and clinicians together consider both the implications of the questions asked and the ways of knowing, exploring, and understanding such phenomena.

References

American Psychiatric Association. (1994). *Diagnostic and statistical manual of mental disorders* (4th ed.). Washington, DC: Author.

American Psychological Association. (1992). Ethical principles of psychologists and code of conduct. *American Psychologist, 47*(12), 1597–1611.

Barclay, C. R. (1986). Schematization of autobiographical memory. In D. C. Rubin (Ed.), *Autobiographical memory* (pp. 82–99). New York: Cambridge University Press.

Barclay, C. R. (1988). Truth and accuracy in autobiographical memory. In M. M. Gruneberg, P. E. Morris, & R. N. Sykes (Eds.), *Practical aspects of memory: Current research and issues: Vol. 1. Memory in everyday life* (pp. 289–294). New York: Wiley.

Barclay, C. R. (1994). Composing protoselves through improvisation. In U. Neisser & R. Fivush (Eds.), *The remembering self: Construction and accuracy in the self-narrative* (pp. 55–77). New York: Cambridge University Press.

Barclay, C. R., & DeCooke, P. A. (1988). Ordinary everyday memories: Some of the things of which selves are made. In U. Neisser & E. Winograd (Eds.), *Remembering reconsidered: Ecological and traditional approaches to the study of memory* (pp. 91–125). New York: Cambridge University Press.

Barsalou, L. W. (1988). The content and organization of autobiographical memories. In U. Neisser & E. Winograd (Eds.), *Remembering reconsidered: Ecological and traditional approaches to the study of memory* (pp. 193–243). New York: Cambridge University Press.

Bartlett, F. C. (1932). *Remembering: A study in experimental and social psychology.* Cambridge, England: Cambridge University Press.

Bauer, P. J. (1995). Recalling past events: From infancy to early childhood. In R. Vasta (Ed.), *Annals of child development* (Vol. 11, pp. 25–71). London: Jessica Kingsley.

Bauer, P. J., Hertsgaard, L. A., & Dow, G. A. (1994). After 8 months have passed: Long-term recall of events by 1- to 2-year old children. *Memory, 2*(4), 353–382.

Bauer, P. J., & Mandler, J. M. (1990). Remembering what happened next: Very young children's recall of event sequences. In R. Fivush & J. A. Hudson (Eds.), *Knowing and remembering in young children* (pp. 9–29). New York: Cambridge University Press.

Beahrs, J. O. (1982). *Unity and multiplicity: Multilevel consciousness of self in hypnosis, psychiatric disorder, and mental health.* New York: Brunner/Mazel.

Berliner, L., & Williams, L. M. (1994). Memories of child sexual abuse: A response to Lindsay and Read. *Applied Cognitive Psychology, 8,* 379–387.

Bonanno, G. A. (1990a). Repression, accessibility, and the translation of private experience. *Psychoanalytic Psychology, 7*(4), 453–473.

Bonanno, G. A. (1990b). Remembering and psychotherapy. *Psychotherapy, 27*(2), 175–186.

Bower, G. H. (1990). Awareness, the unconscious, and repression: An experimental psychologist's perspective. In J. L. Singer (Ed.), *Repression and dissociation: Implications for personality theory, psychopathology, and health* (pp. 209–231). Chicago: University of Chicago Press.

Boyer, M. E., Barron, K. L., & Farrar, M. J. (1994). Three-year-olds remember a novel event from 20 months: Evidence for long-term memory in children? *Memory, 2*(4), 417–445.

Braun, B. G. (1990). Dissociative disorders as sequelae to incest. In R. P. Kluft (Ed.), *Incest-related syndromes of adult psychopathology* (pp. 227–246). Washington DC: American Psychiatric Press.

Bremner, J. D., Davis, M., Southwick, S. M., Krystal, J. H., & Charney, D. S. (1993). Neurobiology of post-traumatic stress disorder. In J. M. Oldman, M. B. Riba, & A. Tasman (Eds.), *American*

Psychiatric Press review of psychiatry (Vol. 12, pp. 183–205). Washington, DC: American Psychiatric Press.

Brewer, W. (1986). What is autobiographical memory? In D. C. Rubin (Ed.), *Autobiographical memory* (pp. 25–49). New York: Cambridge University Press.

Briere, J. (1989). *Therapy for adults molested as children: Beyond survival.* New York: Springer.

Briere, J. (1992). *Child abuse trauma: Theory and treatment of the lasting effects.* Newbury Park, CA: Sage.

Briere, J. (1995). Science versus politics in the delayed memory debate: A commentary. *Counseling Psychologist, 23*(2), 290–293.

Briere, J., & Conte, J. (1993). Self-reported amnesia for abuse in adults molested as children. *Journal of Traumatic Stress, 6*(1), 21–31.

Bruhn, A. R. (1990). *Earliest childhood memories: Vol. 1. Theory and application to clinical practice.* New York: Praeger.

Bruner, J. S. (1964). The course of cognitive growth. *American Psychologist, 19,* 1–15.

Bruner, J. S. (1987). Life as narrative. *Social Research, 54,* 11–32.

Bruner, J. S. (1994). The "remembered" self. In U. Neisser & R. Fivush (Eds.), *The remembering self: Construction and accuracy in the self-narrative* (pp. 41–54). New York: Cambridge University Press.

Burgess, A. W., & Hartman, C. R. (1992). Memory, cognition, and childhood trauma. In A. W. Burgess (Ed.), *Child trauma I: Issues and research* (pp. 61–86). New York: Garland.

Burke, A., Heuer, F., & Reisberg, D. (1992). Remembering emotional events. *Memory and Cognition, 20*(3), 277–290.

Cardeña, E. (1994). The domain of dissociation. In S. J. Lynn & J. W. Rhue (Eds.), *Dissociation: Clinical and theoretical perspectives* (pp. 1–31). New York: Guilford Press.

Carlson, N. R. (1991). *Physiology of behavior* (4th ed.). Boston: Allyn & Bacon.

Ceci, S. J., & Bruck, M. (1993). Suggestibility of the child witness: A historical review and synthesis. *Psychological Bulletin, 113*(3), 403–439.

Ceci, S. J., Huffman, M. L. C., Smith, E., & Loftus, E. F. (1994). Repeatedly thinking about a non-event: Source misattributions among preschoolers. *Consciousness and Cognition, 3,* 388–407.

Ceci, S. J., & Loftus, E. F. (1994). "Memory work": A royal road to false memories? *Applied Cognitive Psychology, 8,* 351–364.

Charney, D. S., Deutch, A. Y., Krystal, J. H., Southwick, S. M., & Davis, M. (1993). Psychobiologic mechanisms of posttraumatic stress disorder. *Archives of General Psychiatry, 50,* 294–305.

Chemtob, C., Roitblat, H. L., Hamada, R. S., Carlson, J. G., & Twentyman, C. T. (1988). A cognitive action theory of post-traumatic stress disorder. *Journal of Anxiety Disorders, 2,* 253–275.

Christianson, S., & Loftus, E. F. (1990). Some characteristics of people's traumatic memories. *Psychonomic Society Bulletin, 28*(3), 195–198.

Christianson, S., & Loftus, E. F. (1991). Remembering emotional events: The fate of detailed information. *Cognition and Emotion, 5*(2), 81–108.

Christianson, S., & Nilsson, L. (1984). Functional amnesia as induced by a psychological trauma. *Memory and Cognition, 12*(2), 142–155.

Christianson, S., & Nilsson, L. (1989). Hysterical amnesia: A case of aversively motivated isolation of memory. In R. Archer & L. Nilsson (Eds.), *Aversion, avoidance, and anxiety: Perspectives on aversively motivated behavior* (pp. 289–310). Hillsdale, NJ: Erlbaum.

Claridge, K. (1992). Reconstructing memories of abuse: A theory-based approach. *Psychotherapy, 29*(1), 243–252.

Courtois, C. A. (1991). Theory, sequencing, and strategy in treating adult survivors. *New Directions for Mental Health Services, 51,* 47–60.

Courtois, C. A. (1992). The memory retrieval process in incest survivor therapy. *Journal of Child Sexual Abuse, 1*(1), 15–31.

Courtois, C. A. (1995). Scientist-practitioners and the delayed memory controversy: Scientific standards and the need for collaboration. *Counseling Psychologist, 23*(2), 294–299.

Curtis, J. C. (1991). Dr. Curtis' response. In J. A. Chu (Ed.), The critical issues task force report: Strategies for evaluating the validity of reports of childhood abuse. *International Society for the Study of Multiple Personality and Dissociation Newsletter, 9*(6), 5–7.

Ellenberger, H. (1970). *The discovery of the unconscious: The history and evolution of dynamic psychiatry.* New York: Basic Books.

Enns, C. A., McNeilly, C. L., Corkery, J. M., & Gilbert, M. S. (1995). The debate about delayed memories of child sexual abuse: A feminist perspective. *Counseling Psychologist, 23*(2), 181–279.

Erdelyi, M. (1990). Repression, reconstruction, and defense: History and integration of the psychoanalytic and experimental frameworks. In J. L. Singer (Ed.), *Repression and dissociation: Implications for personality theory, psychopathology, and health* (pp. 1–32). Chicago: University of Chicago Press.

Erdelyi, M., & Goldberg, B. (1979). Let's not sweep repression under the rug: Toward a cognitive psychology of repression. In J. Kihlstrom & F. J. Evans (Eds.), *Functional disorders of memory* (pp. 355–402). Hillsdale, NJ: Erlbaum.

Eth, S. (1988). The child victim as witness in sexual abuse proceedings. *Psychiatry, 51,* 221–232.

Ewin, D. W. (1994). How memories retrieved with hypnosis are accurate. *American Journal of Clinical Hypnosis, 36*(3), 174–176.

Farrar, M. J., & Goodman, G. S. (1990). Developmental differences in the relation between script and episodic memory: Do they exist? In R. Fivush & J. A. Hudson (Eds.), *Knowing and remembering in young children* (pp. 30–64). New York: Cambridge University Press.

Fine, C. G. (1990). The cognitive sequelae of incest. In R. P. Kluft (Ed.), *Incest-related syndromes of adult psychopathology* (pp. 161–182). Washington, DC: American Psychiatric Press.

Fitzgerald, J. M. (1990). A developmental account of early childhood amnesia. *Journal of Genetic Psychology, 152*(2), 159–171.

Fivush, R. (1991). The social construction of personal narratives. *Merrill–Palmer Quarterly, 37*(1), 59–81.

Fivush, R. (1994a). Introductory comments. *Memory, 2*(4), 337–338.

Fivush, R. (1994b). Young children's event recall: Are memories constructed through discourse? *Consciousness and Cognition, 3,* 356–373.

Fivush, R., Haden, C., & Adam, S. (1995). Structure and coherence of preschooler's personal narratives over time: Implications for childhood amnesia. *Journal of Experimental Child Psychology, 60,* 32–56.

Fivush, R., & Hamond, N. R. (1990). Autobiographical memory across the preschool years: Toward reconceptualizing childhood amnesia. In R. Fivush & J. A. Hudson (Eds.), *Knowing and remembering in young children* (pp. 223–248). New York: Cambridge University Press.

Freud, S. (1892a/1963). Early studies on the psychical mechanism of hysterical phenomena. In P. Rieff (Ed. and Trans.), *Early psychoanalytic writings* (pp. 27–34). New York: Macmillan.

Freud, S. (1892b/1963). On the psychical mechanism of hysterical phenomena. In P. Rieff (Ed. and Trans.), *Early psychoanalytic writings* (pp. 35–50). New York: Macmillan.

Freud, S. (1896/1963). The aetiology of hysteria. In P. Rieff (Ed. and Trans.), *Early psychoanalytic writings* (pp. 175–204). New York: Macmillan.

Freud, S. (1899/1963). Screen memories. In P. Rieff (Ed. and Trans.), *Early psychoanalytic writings* (pp. 229–250). New York: Macmillan.

Freud, S. (1900/1965). The interpretation of dreams. In J. Strachey (Ed. and Trans.), *The standard edition of the complete psychological works of Sigmund Freud* (Vols. 4 and 5). London: Hogarth Press.

Freud, S. (1912/1963). A note on the unconscious in psychoanalysis. In P. Rieff (Ed. and Trans.), *General psychological theory* (pp. 49–55). New York: Collier Books.

Freud, S. (1915a/1963). Repression. In P. Rieff (Ed. and Trans.), *General psychological theory* (pp. 104–115). New York: Collier Books.

Freud, S. (1915b/1963). The unconscious. In P. Rieff (Ed. and Trans.), *General psychological theory* (pp. 116–150). New York: Collier Books.

Freud, S. (1917/1966). *Introductory lectures on psychoanalysis* (J. Strachey, Ed. and Trans.). New York: Norton.

Freud, S. (1938/1964). Splitting of the ego in the process of defence. In J. Strachey (Ed. and Trans.), *The standard edition of the complete psychological works of Sigmund Freud* (Vol. 23, pp. 275–278). London: Hogarth Press.

Fromm, E. (1992). Dissociation, repression, cognition, and voluntarism. *Consciousness and Cognition, 1,* 40–46.

Ganaway, G. K. (1989). Historical versus narrative truth: Clarifying the role of exogenous trauma in the etiology of MPD and its variants. *Dissociation, 2*(4), 205–220.

References

Ganaway, G. K. (1991a, August). *Alternative hypotheses regarding satanic ritual abuse memories.* Paper presented at the annual meeting of the American Psychological Association, San Francisco.

Ganaway, G. K. (1991b). Dr. Ganaway's response. In, J. A. Chu (Ed.), The critical issues task force report: Strategies for evaluating the validity of reports of childhood abuse. *International Society for the Study of Multiple Personality and Dissociation Newsletter, 9*(6), 5–7.

Garry, M., Loftus, E. F., & Brown, S. (1994). Memory: A river runs through it. *Consciousness and Cognition, 3,* 438–451.

Gergen, K. J., & Kaye, J. (1992). Beyond narrative in the negotiation of therapeutic meaning. In S. McNamee & K. J. Gergen (Eds.), *Therapy as social construction* (pp. 166–185). London: Sage.

Goodman G. S., & Golding, J. (1983, April). Effects of real-world knowledge on memory. In K. Nelson (Chair), *Memory and representation of the real world.* Symposium at the Society for Research in Child Development, Detroit, MI.

Goodman, G. S., Hirschman, J. E., Hepps, D., & Rudy, L. (1991). Children's memory for stressful events. *Merrill–Palmer Quarterly, 37*(1), 109–153.

Goodman, G. S., Quas, J. A., Batterman-Faunce, J. M., Riddlesberger, M. M., & Kuhn, J. (1994). Predictors of accurate and inaccurate memories of traumatic events experienced in childhood. *Consciousness and Cognition, 3,* 269–294.

Goodman, G. S., Rudy, L., Bottoms, B. L., & Aman, C. (1990). Children's concerns and memory: Issues of ecological validity in the study of children's eyewitness testimony. In R. Fivush & J. A. Hudson (Eds.), *Knowing and remembering in young children* (pp. 249–284). New York: Cambridge University Press.

Greenberg, M. S., & van der Kolk, B. (1987). Retrieval and integration of traumatic memories with the "painting cure." In B. van der Kolk (Ed.), *Psychological trauma* (pp. 191–216). Washington, DC: American Psychiatric Press.

Greenwald, A. G. (1992). New look 3: Unconscious cognition reclaimed. *American Psychologist, 47*(6), 766–779.

Hall, J. M. (1992, August). *Dissociative reactions to incest.* Paper presented at the annual convention of the American Psychological Association, Washington, DC.

Hartman, C. R., & Burgess, A. W. (1993). Information processing of trauma. *Child Abuse and Neglect, 17,* 47–58.

Harvey, M. R., & Herman, J. L. (1994). Amnesia, partial amnesia, and delayed recall among adult survivors of childhood trauma. *Conscious and Cognition, 3,* 295–306.

Herman, J. L. (1992). *Trauma and recovery.* New York: Basic Books.

Herman, J. L., & Schatzow, E. (1987). Recovery and verification of memories of childhood sexual trauma. *Psychoanalytic Psychology, 4*(1), 1–14.

Hewitt, S. K. (1994). Preverbal sexual abuse: What two children report in later years. *Child Abuse and Neglect, 18*(10), 821–826.

Hilgard, E. R. (1977). *Divided consciousness: Multiple controls in human thought and action.* New York: Wiley.

Hilgard, E. R. (1992). Divided consciousness and dissociation. *Consciousness and Cognition, 1,* 16–31.

Hilgard, E. R. (1994). Neodissociation theory. In S. J. Lynn & J. W. Rhue (Eds.), *Dissociation: Clinical and theoretical perspectives* (pp. 32–51). New York: Guilford Press.

Holmes, D. S. (1990). The evidence for repression: An examination of sixty years of research. In J. L. Singer (Ed.), *Repression and dissociation: Implications for personality, theory, psychopathology, and health* (pp. 85–102). Chicago: University of Chicago Press.

Horowitz, M. J. (1986). *Stress response syndromes.* Northvale, NJ: Jason Aronson.

Horowitz, M. J. (1988). *Introduction to psychodynamics: A new synthesis.* New York: Basic Books.

Horowitz, M. J. (1991). Person schemas. In M. J. Horowitz (Ed.), *Person schemas and maladaptive interpersonal patterns* (pp. 13–32). Chicago: University of Chicago Press.

Horowitz, M. J. (1992). Conscious representation. *Consciousness and Cognition, 1,* 12–15.

Howe, M. L., & Courage, M. L. (1993). On resolving the enigma of infantile amnesia. *Psychological Bulletin, 113*(2), 305–326.

Howe, M. L., Courage, M. L., & Peterson, C. (1994). How can I remember when "I" wasn't there: Long-term retention of traumatic experiences and emergence of the cognitive self. *Consciousness and Cognition, 3,* 327–355.

Howe, M. L., Kelland, A., Bryant-Brown, L., & Clark, S. L. (1992).

Measuring the development of children's amnesia and hypermnesia. In M. L. Howe, C. J. Brainerd, & V. F. Reyna (Eds.), *Development of long-term retention* (pp. 56–102). New York: Springer-Verlag.

Howe, M. L., O'Sullivan, J. T., & Marche, T. A. (1992). Toward a theory of the development of long-term retention. In M. L. Howe, C. J. Brainerd, & V. F. Reyna (Eds.), *Development of long-term retention* (pp. 245–256). New York: Springer-Verlag.

Hudson, J. A. (1986). Memories are made of this: General event knowledge and the development of autobiographical memory. In K. Nelson (Ed.), *Event knowledge: Structure and function in development* (pp. 97–118). Hillsdale, NJ: Erlbaum.

Hudson, J. A. (1990). The emergence of autobiographical memory in mother–child conversation. In R. Fivush & J. A. Hudson (Eds.), *Knowing and remembering in young children* (pp. 166–198). New York: Cambridge University Press.

Hudson, J. A. (1993). Understanding events: The development of script knowledge. In M. Bennett (Ed.), *The development of social cognition: The child as psychologist,* (pp. 142–167). New York: Guilford Press.

Hyde, N. (1990). Voices from the silence: Use of imagery with incest survivors. In T. A. Laidlaw & C. Malmo (Eds.), *Healing voices: Feminist approaches to therapy with women* (pp. 163–193). San Francisco: Jossey-Bass.

Janet, P. (1892/1977). *The mental state of hystericals* (C. R. Corson, Trans.; D. N. Robinson, Ed.). Washington, DC: University Publications of America.

Janoff-Bulman, R. (1989). Assumptive worlds and the stress of traumatic events: Applications of the schema construct. *Social Cognition,* 7(2), 113–136.

Johnson, M. K. (1991). Reflection, reality monitoring, and the self. In R. G. Kunzendorf (Ed.), *Mental imagery* (pp. 3–16). New York: Plenum Press.

Khan, A. U. (1986). *Clinical disorders of memory.* New York: Plenum Press.

Kihlstrom, J. F. (1990). The psychological unconscious. In L. A. Pervin (Ed.), *Handbook of personality: Theory and research* (pp. 445–464). New York: Guilford Press.

Kihlstrom, J. F. (1992). Dissociation and dissociations: A comment on consciousness and cognition. *Consciousness and Cognition, 1,* 16–31.

Kihlstrom, J. F., & Hoyt, I. P. (1990). Repression, dissociation, and hypnosis. In J. L. Singer (Ed.), *Repression and dissociation: Implications for personality theory, psychopathology, and health* (pp. 181–208). Chicago: University of Chicago Press.

Kinston W., & Cohen, J. (1986). Primal repression: Clinical and theoretical aspects. *International Journal of Psycho-Analysis, 67,* 337–355.

Kirschner, L. A. (1993). Concepts of reality and psychic reality in psychoanalysis as illustrated by the disagreement between Freud and Ferenczi. *International Journal of Psycho-Analysis, 74,* 219–230.

Kirschner, S., Kirschner, D. A., & Rappaport, R. L. (1993). *Working with adult incest survivors: The healing journey.* New York: Brunner/Mazel.

Kohut, H. (1971). *The analysis of self.* New York: International Universities Press.

Laub, D., & Auerhahn, N. C. (1993). Knowing and not knowing massive psychic trauma: Forms of traumatic memory. *International Journal of Psycho-Analysis, 74,* 287–302.

Lehman, E. B., & Bovasso, M. (1993). Development of intentional forgetting in children. In M. L. Howe & R. Pasnak (Eds.), *Emerging themes in cognitive development: Vol. I. Foundations* (pp. 214–233). New York: Springer-Verlag.

Leichtman, M. D., & Ceci, S. J. (1993). The problem of infantile amnesia: Lessons from fuzzy-trace theory. In M. L. Howe & R. Pasnak (Eds.), *Emerging themes in cognitive development: Vol. I. Foundations* (pp. 195–213). New York: Springer-Verlag.

Levis, D. J. (1990). The recovery of traumatic memories: The etiological source of psychopathology. In R. G. Kunzendorf (Ed.), *Mental imagery* (pp. 233–240). New York: Plenum Press.

Lindsay, D. S. (1994). Contextualizing and clarifying criticisms of memory work in psychotherapy. *Consciousness and Cognition, 3,* 426–437.

Lindsay, D. S. (1995). Beyond backlash: Comments on Enns, McNeilly, Corkery, and Gilbert. *Counseling Psychologist, 23*(2), 280–289.

Lindsay, D. S., & Read, J. D. (1994). Psychotherapy and memories of childhood sexual abuse: A cognitive perspective. *Applied Cognitive Psychology, 8,* 281–338.

Liwag, M. D., & Stein, N. L. (1995). Children's memory for emotional events: The importance of emotion-related retrieval cues. *Journal of Experimental Child Psychology, 60,* 2–31.

Loftus, E. F. (1979). The malleability of human memory. *American Scientist, 67*(3), 312–320.

Loftus, E. F. (1993). The reality of repressed memories. *American Psychologist, 48*(5), 518–537.

Loftus, E. F. (1994). Memories of childhood sexual abuse: Remembering and repressing. *Psychology of Women Quarterly, 18,* 67–84.

Loftus, E. F., & Christianson, S. (1989). Malleability of memory for emotional events. In R. Archer & L. Nilsson (Eds.), *Aversion, avoidance, and anxiety: Perspectives on aversively motivated behavior* (pp. 311–322). Hillsdale, NJ: Erlbaum.

Loftus, E. F., Garry, M., & Feldman, J. (1994). Forgetting sexual trauma: What does it mean when 38% forget? *Journal of Consulting and Clinical Psychology, 62*(6), 1177–1181.

Loftus, E. F., Hoffman, H. G., & Wagenaar, W. A. (1992). The misinformation effect: Transformations in memory induced by postevent information. In M. L. Howe, C. J. Brainerd, & V. F. Reyna (Eds.), *Development of long-term retention* (pp. 159–183). New York: Springer-Verlag

Loftus, E. F., & Kaufman, L. (1992). Why do traumatic experiences sometimes produce good memory (flashbulbs) and sometimes no memory (repression)? In E. Winograd & U. Neisser (Eds.), *Affect and accuracy in recall: Studies of "flashbulb" memories* (pp. 212–223). New York: Cambridge University Press.

Loftus, E. F., & Loftus, G. R. (1980). On the permanence of stored information in the human brain. *American Psychologist, 35*(5), 409–420.

Loftus, E. F., Milo, E. M., & Paddock, J. R. (1995). The accidental executioner: Why psychotherapy must be informed by science. *Counseling Psychologist, 23*(2), 300–309.

MacKay, D. G. (1988). Practical applications and theories of memory: A new epistemiology to supplement the old. In M. M. Gruneberg, P. E. Morris, & R. N. Sykes (Eds.), *Practical aspects of memory:*

Current research and issues: Vol. 2. Clinical and educational implications (pp. 441–446). New York: Wiley.

Malmo, C. (1990). Recovering the past: Using hypnosis to heal childhood trauma survivors. In T. A. Laidlaw & C. Malmo (Eds.), *Healing voices: Feminist approaches to therapy with women* (pp. 194–220). San Francisco: Jossey-Bass.

Mandler, J. M. (1983). Representation. In J. H. Flavell & M. Markman (Eds.), *Manual of child psychology: Vol. 3. Cognitive development* (pp. 420–494). New York: Wiley.

Mandler, J. M. (1990). Recall and its verbal expression. In R. Fivush & J. A. Hudson (Eds.), *Knowing and remembering in young children* (pp. 317–331). New York: Cambridge University Press.

McCann, I. L., & Pearlman, L. A. (1990). *Psychological trauma and the adult survivor: Theory, therapy, and transformation.* New York: Brunner/Mazel.

McDonough, L., & Mandler, J. M. (1994). Very long-term recall in infants: Infantile amnesia reconsidered. *Memory, 2*(4), 339–352.

McGaugh, J. L., Introini-Collison, I. B., Naghara, A. H., & Cahill, L. (1989). Involvement of the amygdala in hormonal and neurotransmitter interactions in the modulation of memory storage. In R. Archer & L. Nilsson (Eds.), *Aversion, avoidance, and anxiety: Perspectives on aversively motivated behavior* (pp. 231–250). Hillsdale, NJ: Erlbaum.

McNally, R. J. (1993). Self-representation in post-traumatic stress disorder: A cognitive perspective. In Z. V. Segal & S. J. Blatt (Eds.), *The self in emotional distress: Cognitive and psychodynamic perspectives* (pp. 71–91). New York: Guilford Press.

Meltzoff, A. N. (1995). What infant memory tells us about infantile amnesia: Long-term recall and deferred imitation. *Journal of Experimental Child Psychology, 59,* 497–515.

Morris, H. (1993). Narrative representation, narrative enactment, and the psychoanalytic construction of history. *International Journal of Psycho-Analysis, 74,* 33–54.

Murray, S. (1988). Cross-modal integration in children's memory. In M. M. Gruneberg, P. E. Morris, R. N. Sykes (Eds.), *Practical aspects of memory: Current research and issues: Vol. 2. Clinical and educational implications* (pp. 281–286). New York: Wiley.

Myers, N. A., Perris, E. E., & Speaker, C. J. (1994). Fifty months of memory: A longitudinal study in early childhood. *Memory, 2(4)*, 383–415.

Neimeyer, G. J., & Metzler, A. E. (1994). Personal identity and auto-biographical recall. In U. Neisser & R. Fivush (Eds.), *The remembering self: Construction and accuracy in the self-narrative* (pp. 105–135). New York: Cambridge University Press.

Neisser, U. (1986). Nested structure in autobiographical memory. In D. C. Rubin (Ed.), *Autobiographical memory* (pp. 71–82). New York: Cambridge University Press.

Neisser, U. (1988). What is ordinary memory the memory of? In U. Neisser & E. Winograd (Eds.), *Remembering reconsidered: Ecological and traditional approaches to the study of memory* (pp. 356–373). New York: Cambridge University Press.

Neisser, U. (1990). Learning from the children. In R. Fivush & J. A. Hudson (Eds.), *Knowing and remembering in young children* (pp. 331–346). New York: Cambridge University Press.

Neisser, U. (1994). Self-narratives: True and false. In U. Neisser & R. Fivush (Eds.), *The remembering self: Construction and accuracy in the self-narrative* (pp. 1–18). New York: Cambridge University Press.

Nelson, K. (1988). The ontogeny of memory for real events. In U. Neisser & E. Winograd (Eds.), *Remembering reconsidered: Ecological and traditional approaches to the study of memory* (pp. 244–282). New York: Cambridge University Press.

Nelson, K. (1990). Remembering, forgetting, and childhood amnesia. In R. Fivush & J. A. Hudson (Eds.), *Knowing and remembering in young children* (pp. 301–317). New York: Cambridge University Press.

Nelson, K. (1993). The psychological and social origins of autobiographical memory. *Psychological Science, 4(1)*, 7–14.

Nelson, K. (1994). Long-term retention of memory for preverbal experience: Evidence and implications. *Memory, 2(4)*, 467–475.

Nemiah, J. C. (1979). Dissociative amnesia: A clinical and theoretical reconsideration. In J. Kihlstrom & F. J. Evans (Eds.), *Functional disorders of memory* (pp. 303–323). Hillsdale, NJ: Erlbaum.

Nurcombe, B. (1986). The child as witness: Competency and credibility. *Journal of the American Academy of Child Psychiatry, 25(4)*, 473–480.

Ornstein, P. A., Gordon, B. N., & Baker-Ward, L. E. (1992). Children's memory for salient events: Implications for testimony. In M. L. Howe, C. J. Brainerd, & V. F. Reyna (Eds.), *Development of long-term retention* (pp. 135–158). New York: Springer-Verlag.

Parkin, A. J. (1987). *Memory and amnesia: An introduction*. Oxford, England: Basil Blackwell.

Pervin, L. A. (1990). Personality theory and research: Prospects for the future. In L. A. Pervin (Ed.), *Handbook of personality: Theory and research* (pp.723–727). New York: Guilford Press.

Pezdek, K. (1994). The illusion of illusory memory. *Applied Cognitive Psychology, 8,* 339–350.

Pezdek, K., & Roe, C. (1994). Memory for childhood events: How suggestible is it? *Consciousness and Cognition, 3,* 374–387.

Pezdek, K., & Roe, C. (1995). The effect of memory trace strength on suggestibility. *Journal of Experimental Child Psychology, 60,* 116–128.

Piaget, J. (1962). *Play, dreams, and imitation in childhood*. New York: Norton.

Piaget, J. (1969). *The child's conception of time*. New York: Ballantine Books.

Piaget, J. (1970). *Structuralism*. New York: Basic Books.

Pillemer, D. B., & White, S. H. (1989). Childhood events recalled by children and adults. In H. N. Reese (Ed.), *Advances in child development and behavior* (Vol. 21, pp. 297–340). San Diego: Academic Press.

Pitman, R. K. (1989). Post-traumatic stress disorder, hormones, and memory. *Biological Psychiatry, 26,* 221–223.

Putnam, F. W. (1989). Pierre Janet and modern views of dissociation. *Journal of Traumatic Stress, 2*(4), 413–429.

Putnam, F. W. (1990). Disturbances of "self" in victims of childhood sexual abuse. In R. P. Kluft (Ed.), *Incest-related syndromes of adult psychopathology* (pp. 113–132). Washington, DC: American Psychiatric Press.

Putnam, F. W. (1991). Dissociative phenomena. In A. Tasman & S. M. Goldfinger (Eds.), *American Psychiatric Press review of psychiatry* (Vol. 10, pp. 145–160). Washington, DC: American Psychiatric Press.

Putnam, F. W. (1993). Dissociative disorders in children: Behavioral profiles and problems. *Child Abuse and Neglect, 17,* 39–45.

Pynoos, R. S., & Eth, S. (1985). Developmental perspectives on psychic trauma in childhood. In C. R. Figley (Ed.), *Trauma and its wake: The study and treatment of post-traumatic stress disorder* (pp. 36–52). New York: Brunner/Mazel.

Pynoos, R. S., & Nader, K. (1989). Children's memory and proximity to violence. *Journal of the American Academy of Child and Adolescent Psychiatry, 28*(2), 236–241.

Ratner, H. H., Smith, B. S., & Padgett, R. J. (1990). Children's organization of events and event memories. In R. Fivush & J. A. Hudson (Eds.), *Knowing and remembering in young children* (pp. 65–93). New York: Cambridge University Press.

Read, J. D., & Lindsay, D. S. (1994). Moving toward a middle ground on the "false memory debate": Reply to commentaries on Lindsay and Read. *Applied Cognitive Psychology, 8,* 407–435.

Reyna, V. F. (1992). Reasoning, remembering, and their relationship: Social, cognitive, and developmental issues. In M. L. Howe, C. J. Brainerd, & V. F. Reyna (Eds.), *Development of long-term retention* (pp. 103–132). New York: Springer-Verlag.

Rovee-Collier, C., & Shyi, C.-W. G. (1992). A functional and cognitive analysis of infant long-term retention. In M. L. Howe, C. J. Brainerd, & V. F. Reyna (Eds.), *Development of long-term retention* (pp. 3–55). New York: Springer-Verlag.

Schachtel, E. G. (1947/1982). On memory and childhood amnesia. In U. Neisser (Ed.), *Memory observed: Remembering in natural contexts* (pp. 189–200). San Francisco: Freeman.

Schachtel, E. G. (1959). *Metamorphosis: On the development of affect, perception, attention, and memory.* New York: Basic Books.

Schacter, D. L., Kihlstrom, J. F., Kihlstrom, L. C., & Berren, M. B. (1989). Autobiographical memory in a case of multiple personality disorder. *Journal of Abnormal Psychology, 98*(4), 508–513.

Schetky, D. H. (1990). A review of the literature on the long-term effects of childhood sexual abuse. In R. P. Kluft (Ed.), *Incest-related syndromes of adult psychopathology* (pp. 35–54). Washington, DC: American Psychiatric Press.

Sheffield, E. G., & Hudson, J. A. (1994). Reactivation of toddlers' event memory. *Memory, 2*(4), 447–465.

Singer, J. A., & Salovey, P. (1993). *The remembered self: Emotion and memory in personality.* New York: Free Press.

Singer, J. L., & Salovey, P. (1991). Organized knowledge structures and personality. In M. J. Horowitz (Ed.), *Person schemas and maladaptive interpersonal patterns* (pp. 33–80). Chicago: University of Chicago Press.

Singer, J. L., & Sincoff, J. B. (1990). Summary: Beyond repression and the defenses. In J. L. Singer (Ed.), *Repression and dissociation: Implications for personality theory, psychopathology, and health* (pp. 471–496). Chicago: University of Chicago Press.

Spence, D. P. (1982). *Narrative truth and historical truth: Meaning and interpretation in psychoanalysis.* New York: Norton.

Spiegel, D. (1990). Trauma, dissociation, and hypnosis. In R. P. Kluft (Ed.), *Incest-related syndromes of adult psychopathology* (pp. 247–262). Washington DC: American Psychiatric Press.

Spiegel, D., Frishholz, E. J., & Spira, J. (1993). Functional disorders of memory. In J. M. Oldham, M. B. Riba, & A. Tasman (Eds.), *American Psychiatric Press review of psychiatry* (Vol. 12, pp. 747–782). Washington, DC: American Psychiatric Press.

Stinson, C. H., & Palmer, S. E. (1991). Parallel distributed processing models of person schemas and psychopathologies. In M. J. Horowitz (Ed.), *Person schemas and maladaptive interpersonal patterns* (pp. 339–378). Chicago: University of Chicago Press.

Sugar, M. (1992). Toddler's traumatic memories. *Infant Mental Health Journal, 13*(3), 245–251.

Swanson, J. M., & Kinsbourne, M. (1979). State dependent learning and retrieval: Methodological cautions and theoretical considerations. In J. F. Kihlstrom & F. J. Evans (Eds.), *Functional disorders of memory* (pp. 275–276). Hillsdale, NJ: Analytic Press.

Terr, L. (1983). Chowchilla revisited: The effects of psychic trauma four years after a school-bus kidnapping. *American Journal of Psychiatry, 140*(12), 1543–1550.

Terr, L. (1988). What happens to early memories of trauma? A study of twenty children under age five at the time of documented traumatic events. *Journal of the American Academy of Child and Adolescent Psychiatry, 27*(1), 96–104.

Terr, L. (1990). *Too scared to cry: Psychic trauma in childhood.* New York: Basic Books.

Terr, L. (1991). Childhood traumas: An outline and overview. *American Journal of Psychiatry, 148*(1), 10–20.

Terr, L. (1994). *Unchained memories: True stories of traumatic memories, lost and found.* New York: Basic Books.

Tessler, M., & Nelson, K. (1994). Making memories: The influence of joint encoding on later recall by young children. *Consciousness and Cognition, 3,* 307–326.

Toglia, M. P., Ross, D. F., Ceci, S. J., & Hembrooke, J. (1992). The suggestibility of children's memory: A social-psychological and cognitive interpretation. In M. L. Howe, C. J. Brainerd, & V. F. Reyna (Eds.), *Development of long-term retention* (pp. 217–244). New York: Springer-Verlag.

Tulving, E. (1984). Precis of elements of episodic memory. *Behavioral and Brain Sciences, 7,* 223–268.

Tulving, E. (1985). Memory and consciousness. *Canadian Psychology, 26*(1), 1–12.

Turner, J. (1990). Let my soul soar: Touch therapy. In T. A. Laidlaw & C. Malmo (Eds.), *Healing voices: Feminist approaches to therapy with women* (pp. 221–240). San Francisco: Jossey-Bass.

Ulman, R. B., & Brothers, D. (1988). *The shattered self: A psychoanalytic study of trauma.* Hillsdale, NJ: Analytic Press.

Vaillant, G. E. (1990). Repression in college men followed for half a century. In J. L. Singer (Ed.), *Repression and dissociation: Implications for personality theory, psychopathology, and health* (pp. 259–274). Chicago: University of Chicago Press.

van der Hart, O., Brown, P., & van der Kolk, B. (1989). Pierre Janet's treatment of post-traumatic stress. *Journal of Traumatic Stress, 2*(4), 379–395.

van der Hart, O., & Friedman, B. (1989). A reader's guide to Pierre Janet on dissociation: A neglected intellectual heritage. *Dissociation, 2*(1), 3–16.

van der Kolk, B. (1987). The drug treatment of post-traumatic stress disorder. *Journal of Affective Disorders, 13,* 203–213.

van der Kolk, B., Boyd, H., Krystal, J., & Greenberg, M. (1984). Post-traumatic stress disorder as a biologically based disorder: Implications of the animal model of inescapable shock. In B. van der Kolk (Ed.), *Post-traumatic stress disorder: Psychological and biological sequelae* (pp. 123–134). Washington, DC: American Psychiatric Press.

van der Kolk, B., Brown, P., & van der Hart, O. (1989). Pierre Janet on post-traumatic stress. *Journal of Traumatic Stress, 2*(4), 365–378.

van der Kolk, B., & Greenberg, M. (1987). The psychobiology of the trauma response: Hyperarousal, constriction, and addiction to traumatic reexposure. In B. van der Kolk (Ed.), *Psychological trauma* (pp. 63–88). Washington, DC: American Psychiatric Press.

van der Kolk, B., & Kadish, W. (1987). Amnesia, dissociation, and the return of the repressed. In B. van der Kolk (Ed.), *Psychological trauma* (pp. 173–190). Washington, DC: American Psychiatric Press.

van der Kolk, B., & van der Hart, O. (1989). Pierre Janet and the breakdown of adaptation in psychological trauma. *American Journal of Psychiatry, 146*(12), 1530–1540.

van der Kolk, B., & van der Hart, O. (1991). The intrusive past: The flexibility of memory and the engraving of trauma. *American Imago, 48*(4), 425–454.

Waites, E. A. (1993). *Trauma and survival: Post-traumatic and dissociative disorders in women.* New York: Norton.

Waldvogel, S. (1948/1982). Childhood memories. In U. Neisser (Ed.), *Memory observed: Remembering in natural contexts* (pp. 73–76). San Francisco: Freeman.

Warren, A. R., & Swartwood, J. N. (1992). Developmental issues in flashbulb memory research: Children recall the Challenger event. In E. Winograd & U. Neisser (Eds.), *Affect and accuracy in recall: Studies of "flashbulb" memories* (pp. 95–120). New York: Cambridge University Press.

Weinberger, D. A. (1990). The construct validity of the repressive coping style. In J. L. Singer (Ed.), *Repression and dissociation: Implications for personality theory, psychopathology, and health* (pp. 337–386). Chicago: University of Chicago Press.

Weiser, J. (1990). More than meets the eye: Using ordinary snapshots as tools for therapy. In T. A. Laidlaw & C. Malmo (Eds.), *Healing voices: Feminist approaches to therapy with women* (pp. 83–117). San Francisco: Jossey-Bass.

Wetzler, S. E., & Sweeney, J. A. (1986). Childhood amnesia: An empirical demonstration. In D. C. Rubin (Ed.), *Autobiographical memory* (pp. 191–201). New York: Cambridge University Press.

White, S. H., & Pillemer, D. B. (1979). Childhood amnesia and the development of a socially accessible memory system. In J. F. Kihlstrom & F. J. Evans (Eds.), *Functional disorders of memory* (pp. 29–73). Hillsdale, NJ: Erlbaum.

Williams, L. M. (1994a). Recall of childhood trauma: A prospective study of women's memories of child sexual abuse. *Journal of Consulting and Clinical Psychology, 62*(6), 1167–1176.

Williams, L. M. (1994b). What does it mean to forget child sexual abuse? A reply to Loftus, Garry, and Feldman (1994). *Journal of Consulting and Clinical Psychology, 62*(6), 1182–1186.

Wilson, J. (1989). *Trauma, transformation, and healing.* New York: Brunner/Mazel.

Winnicott, D. W. (1965). *The maturational process and the facilitating environment.* New York: International Universities Press.

Winograd, E. (1988). Continuities between ecological and laboratory approaches to memory. In U. Neisser & E. Winograd (Eds.), *Remembering reconsidered: Ecological and traditional approaches to the study of memory* (pp. 11–20). New York: Cambridge University Press.

Woody, E. Z., & Bowers, K. S. (1994). A frontal assault on dissociated control. In S. J. Lynn & J. W. Rhue (Eds.), *Dissociation: Clinical and theoretical perspectives* (pp. 52–79). New York: Guilford Press.

Zaragoza, M. S., Dahlgren, D., & Muench, J. (1992). The role of memory impairment in children's suggestibility. In M. L. Howe, C. J. Brainerd, & V. F. Reyna (Eds.), *Development of long-term retention* (pp. 184–216). New York: Springer-Verlag.

Author Index

Subject Index